PYRANTEL PARASITICIDE THERAPY IN HUMANS AND DOMESTIC ANIMALS

PYRANTEL PARASITICIDE THERAPY IN HUMANS AND DOMESTIC ANIMALS

Edited by

ALAN A. MARCHIONDO
Adobe Veterinary Parasitology Consulting LLC, Santa Fe, NM,
United States
Retired, Zoetis, Kalamazoo, MI, United States

AMSTERDAM • BOSTON • HEIDELBERG • LONDON
NEW YORK • OXFORD • PARIS • SAN DIEGO
SAN FRANCISCO • SINGAPORE • SYDNEY • TOKYO
Academic Press is an imprint of Elsevier

Academic Press is an imprint of Elsevier
125 London Wall, London EC2Y 5AS, UK
525 B Street, Suite 1800, San Diego, CA 92101-4495, USA
50 Hampshire Street, 5th Floor, Cambridge, MA 02139, USA
The Boulevard, Langford Lane, Kidlington, Oxford OX5 1GB, UK

British Library Cataloguing-in-Publication Data
A catalogue record for this book is available from the British Library

Library of Congress Cataloging-in-Publication Data
A catalog record for this book is available from the Library of Congress

ISBN: 978-0-12-801449-3

For Information on all Academic Press publications
visit our website at http://www.elsevier.com/

Publisher: Sara Tenney
Acquisition Editor: Linda Versteeg-Buschman
Editorial Project Manager: Halima Williams
Production Project Manager: Edward Taylor
Designer: Matthew Limbert

Typeset by MPS Limited, Chennai, India

CONTENTS

LIST OF CONTRIBUTORS

T.G. Geary
Institute of Parasitology, McGill University, St. Anne de Bellevue, QC, Canada

B. Levecke
Laboratory of Parasitology, Ghent University, Merelbeke, Belgium

C.D. Mackenzie
Department of Pathobiology and Diagnostic Investigation, Michigan State University, East Lansing, MI, United States

A.A. Marchiondo
Adobe Veterinary Parasitology Consulting LLC, Santa Fe, NM, United States; Retired, Zoetis, Kalamazoo, MI, United States

R.J. Martin
Department of Biomedical Sciences, College of Veterinary Medicine, Iowa State University, Ames, IA, United States

C.R. Reinemeyer
East Tennessee Clinical Research, Inc., Rockwood, TN, United States

D.J. Sheehan
Zoetis, Kalamazoo, MI, United States

S.M. Sheehan
Zoetis, Kalamazoo, MI, United States

J. Vercruysse
Ghent University Global Campus, Incheon Global Campus Foundation, Incheon, South Korea

PREFACE

Pyrantel and its various salt forms, members of the tetrahydropyrimidine family of compounds (oxantel, morantel), were introduced to the marketplace in the 1970s as veterinary antiparasitic drugs and later in human medicine. Their broad-spectrum of anthelmintic activity against roundworms and hookworms, along with their safety in animals and humans, yielded targeted nematocidal therapeutics with global acceptance and commercial success in single and combination therapies against helminth infections. The inspiration for this book was to (1) capture historical information on the discovery of the tetrahydropyrimidines, lest this information be lost over time, and (2) to provide an up-to-date, comprehensive reference guide on the mode of action, pharmacology, safety, and clinical uses of the tetrahydropyrimidines to control certain helminth infections in domestic animals and humans.

The target audience of this book is not only the basic researcher in antiparasitics and the field researcher involved in parasite control, but also the practicing veterinarian and physician. My hope is that the volume will be useful to advanced undergraduates, graduate students, university and industrial research workers, and teachers in biology, the health sciences, veterinary, and human medicine, as well as veterinarians and physicians.

I am indebted and express my appreciation to each of the authors, considered to be most knowledgeable in the field for their particular chapter contribution, for their thorough reviews, cooperation in meeting deadlines, and in the revision of the manuscripts. However, it must not be inferred that these experts endorse all the views expressed in this book, particularly the chapter on Potential Applications of Tetrahydropyrimidines to Address Unmet Needs. I particularly extend thanks to Halima Williams, Editorial Project Manager, Academic Press/ Elsevier, San Diego, CA, for support and assistance in the publication of the book; to Linda Versteeg, Acquisition Editor, Elsevier, Inc. for her encouragement and enthusiasm for this book; to Richard O. Nicholas, Zoetis, for the extensive literature review; to Bert Baker and Kathryn I. Adamson, Zoetis, for providing answers to regulatory and registration inquiries on some of the end-use products; and especially to Vasillios J. Theodorides, one of the inventors of pyrantel and the sole surviving member of the discovery team, for sharing his experience and perspectives on the discovery of the tetrahydropyrimidines. In a comprehensive review of this kind it is probably inevitable that some errors and omissions will have crept in, in spite of careful checking. The literature on the Tetrahydropyrimidines consists of approximately 4045 citations, thus it was necessary to focus on the relevant literature of the chapter headings.

Respectfully,
Alan A. Marchiondo
December 1, 2015

INTRODUCTION

Prior to the discovery of the Tetrahydropyrimidines, and even today, the prominent trend in chemotherapy and management of parasitic diseases has been the continual search for more effective, broader spectrum, and safer new drugs that could provide marked advances in the field of parasite control [1,2]. Many older drugs used for helminth parasite removal were plant/herbal products or animal and mineral sources used since ancient times, the value of which had been inadequately assessed by clinical observations. Experience with this multitude of remedies supports the old adage that "where there are many cures, there are no cures."

Significant progress in the discovery of antinematodal drugs with insecticide/fungicide activities occurred in the early 1940s (phenothiazine) and early 1960s (thiabendazole), with both drugs possessing medium-spectrum activity in the control of gastrointestinal parasitism. Critical tests of phenothiazine in cattle at 600 mg/kg proved satisfactory against *Haemonchus contortus*, *Trichostrongylus axei*, and *Oesophagostomum radiatum*, but exhibited low efficacies against *Bunostomum phlebotomum* and *Cooperia* spp. and variable activity (75%) against *Ostertagia* spp. [3—5]. Thiabendazole in cattle at the use dosage of 45 mg/kg was shown to be efficacious against adult and L_4 *H. contortus*, *O. ostertagi*, and *T. colubriformis*, but variable in efficacy against adult *Cooperia* spp. [6—8]. The low and variable efficacies of these early anthelmintics spurred the search by scientists at pharmaceutical companies for compounds that would be effective at increasing potencies against all species and all stages of animal nematodes in domestic animals. Since the early 1960s, great strides have been made in the discovery and development of an ideal anthelmintic, resulting in the use of the broad-spectrum antinematodal drugs (imidazoles, tetrahydropyrimidines, macrocyclic lactones, and amino-acetonitrile derivatives).

The majority of new chemical entities introduced, particularly in parasitology, do not originate from de novo design but, rather, are the products of evolution by exploiting existing related chemicals or classes of compounds (ie, the systematic process of changing established structures with established biological properties with the intention of improving the profile of the biological properties) [9]. The chemical evolution approach is driven by empirical screening of a more or less random selection of chemicals to relevant in vitro and in vivo tests in the hope of finding useful biological properties in a novel chemical; that is, lead identification compounds [9]. The chances of success in the identification of a lead compound depend upon the number and structural variety of the compounds screened and the reliability and relevance of the screening tests [9]. Identified leads are then optimized via structure−activity relationship information on the chemicals, the extension of this information to a group of related compounds, and the subsequent arrival at a drug candidate with optimal properties. The processes involved in lead identification and optimization are not to be taken lightly, and involve more failures than successes. Whole parasite in vitro screening followed by in vivo confirmation and spectrum of activity validation has been most valuable in the discovery of new anthelmintics and has led to the discovery of all currently available anthelmintics [10,11].

The discovery of the Tetrahydropyrimidines provides an early example of parasiticide lead identification and optimization using novel in vivo rodent screens followed by confirmation tests against target parasites within host species [12,13]. Close and competitive collaboration between medicinal chemists and parasitologists yielded a highly successful outcome. Identification of the laboratory anthelmintic spectrums of activity of pyrantel, morantel, and oxantel rapidly led to the development and commercialization of products for the treatment and control of nematode infections in animals and humans.

This book contains six chapters on the Tetrahydropyrimidines and begins with this introductory section that sets the stage for the content that follows. The first chapter examines the history of the discovery of the pyrantel chemistry and its salts with details of the chemists and parasitologists in Sandwich, England and in the United States at Groton, CT and Terra Haute, IN involved in the invention. In addition, this section covers the rationale of the chemistry, the structure−activity relationship, and the in vitro and in vivo screens used to determine the activity. The second chapter focuses on the pharmacology of the compounds with known mode of action, the knowledge of existing and potential anthelmintic resistance to this class as it relates to animal health, and the relationships with other anthelmintics that lead to combination anthelmintic therapy. The third chapter explores the known safety of the class in humans and animals based on the pharmacology of the tetrahydropyrimidine class. The fourth chapter provides a listing of the various formulations and devices commercially developed for target animal species in animal health with their spectrum of anthelmintic activity alone, and in combination with other anthelmintics. This section includes subsections by host (dogs, cats, swine, horses, and cattle). The fifth chapter provides an up-to-date review of the use of tetrahydropyrimidines in human medicine globally with indications for therapy, the advantages of this class of anthelmintic, and the current status of anthelmintic resistance mechanisms of the class. Included are strategies to delay anthelmintic resistance in human health. The sixth and final chapter explores potential applications to address unmet needs the class might provide in the future.

Alan A. Marchiondo[1,2]
[1]Adobe Veterinary Parasitology Consulting LLC,
Santa Fe, NM, United States
[2]Retired, Zoetis, Kalamazoo, MI, United States

REFERENCES

[1] Geary TG, Conder GA, Bishop B. The changing landscape of antiparasitic drug discovery for veterinary medicine. Trends Parasitol 2004;20(10):449—55.
[2] Woods DJ, Knauer CS. Veterinary antiparasitic agents in the 21st century: a review from industry. Int J Parasitol 2010;40:1177—81.
[3] Swanson LE, Porter DA, Connelly JW. Efficacy of non-conditioned phenothiazine in removing worms from the alimentary canal of cattle. J Am Vet Med Assoc 1940;96:704—7.
[4] Cauthen GE. The toxic effect of phenothiazine in cattle of the Gulf Coastal plain area of Texas, and its efficacy in removing *Ostertagia ostertagi* and *Trichostrongylus axei*. Am J Vet Res 1953;14:30—2.
[5] Herlich H, Douvres FW, Stewart TB. Trials with phenothiazine variously administered to cattle. Vet Med 1954;49:503—5.
[6] Ames ER, Cheney JM, Rubin R. The efficacy of thiabendazole and bephenium hydroxynaphthoate against *Ostertagi ostertagi* and *Cooperia oncophora* in experimentally infected calves. Am J Vet Res 1963;24:295—9.
[7] Enigk K, Eckert J. Versuche zur Behandlung des Trichostrongylidenbefalls des Rindes mit Thiabendazole. Dtsch tierärztl Wschr [English summary] 1963;70:6—13.
[8] Rubin R, Ames ER, Cheney JM. The efficacy of thiabendazole against *Cooperia oncophora*, *Cooperia punctata*, and *Ostertagia ostertagi* in cattle. Am J Vet Res 1965;26:668—72.
[9] Freter KR. Drug discovery—today and tomorrow: the role of medicinal chemistry. Pharm Res 1988;5(7):397—400.
[10] Campbell WC. Ivermectin, an antiparasitic agent. Med Res Rev 1993;13:61—79.
[11] Geary TG, Sangster NC, Thompson DP. Frontiers in anthelmintic pharmacology. Vet Parasitol 1999;84(3-4):275—95.
[12] Austin WC, Courtney W, Danilewicz JC, Morgan DH, Conover LH, Howes Jr HL, et al. Pyrantel tartrate, a new anthelmintic effective against infections of domestic animals. Nature 1966;212:1273—4.
[13] Howes Jr HL, Lynch JE. Anthelmintic studies with pyrantel. I. Therapeutic and prophylactic efficacy against the enteral stages of various helminths in mice and dogs. J Parasitol 1967;53(5):1085—91.

CHAPTER 1

Discovery and Chemistry of Pyrantel, Morantel and Oxantel

D.J. Sheehan[1], S.M. Sheehan[1] and A.A. Marchiondo[2,3]
[1]Zoetis, Kalamazoo, MI, United States
[2]Adobe Veterinary Parasitology Consulting LLC, Santa Fe, NM, United States
[3]Retired, Zoetis, Kalamazoo, MI, United States

1.1 INTRODUCTION

The discovery of pyrantel (**1**), morantel (**2**), and oxantel (**3**) can only be put into context by defining the history and organization of Pfizer Central Research and the key scientists in medicinal chemistry and parasitology responsible for the research (Fig. 1.1).

The Charles Pfizer & Company was started in 1849 in Williamsburg, Brooklyn by the partnership of the German-American cousins, Charles Pfizer, a chemist, and Charles Erhart, a confectioner, who emigrated from Ludwigsburg, Germany [1]. The company was started as a manufacturer of bulk chemicals such as iodine, boric, tartaric, and citric acids, the latter used for soft drink companies, and produced a wide range of industrial and pharmaceutical products, including the antiparasitic called Santonin (**4**) for the treatment of the human roundworm, *Ascaris lumbricoides* (Fig. 1.2).

In 1919, Pfizer developed expertise in fermentation technology originally for citric acid production and then penicillin during World War II. In 1950, Pfizer discovered and commercialized Terramycin (oxytetracycline, **5**) changing the company from a manufacturer of fine chemicals to a research-based pharmaceutical company with the implementation of a drug discovery program. Terramycin spurred the entry of Pfizer into the animal health industry with the formation of Pfizer's Agricultural Division in the early 1950s and the commercialization of Terramycin-based feed supplements for swine, cattle, and chickens (Fig. 1.3).

Three Pfizer research centers were key to the discovery of pyrantel. In 1952, a 700-acre (2.8 km^2) Agricultural Research Department was established at Terre Haute, Indiana, for the fermentation of streptomycin and Terramycin, along with veterinary facilities to study livestock and poultry diseases. In 1960, Pfizer moved its medical research laboratory and

Pyrantel Parasiticide Therapy in Humans and Domestic Animals.
DOI: http://dx.doi.org/10.1016/B978-0-12-801449-3.00012-0

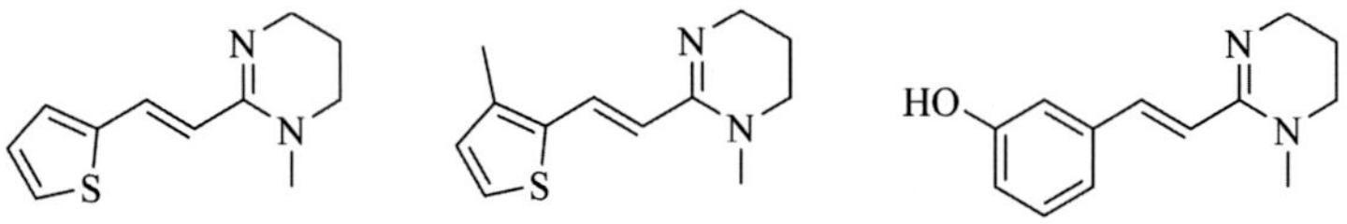

Pyrantel **1** Morantel **2** Oxantel **3**

Figure 1.1 Pyrantel (**1**), Morantel (**2**) and Oxantel (**3**).

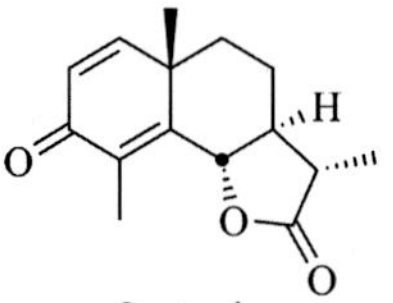

Santonin
4

Figure 1.2 Santonin (**4**).

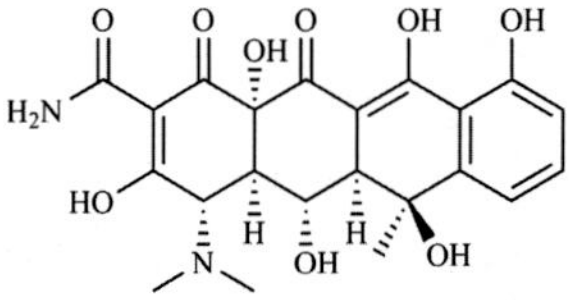

Terramycin
5

Figure 1.3 Terramycin (**5**).

discovery screening out of New York City to a new facility in Groton, Connecticut. Pfizer established operations in the United Kingdom in 1954 on an 80-acre site on the outskirts of Sandwich, Kent [2]. The Agricultural Division opening at the Sandwich site in 1957 was followed by the acquisition by Pfizer of additional land adjacent to its existing site in Sandwich to yield a 390-acre research center in 1964 [3].

Chemical compounds were synthesized and screened in the mid-1960s in a research program carried out by Pfizer's Chemotherapy Research Department and Parasitology Research Department in Sandwich, Kent in collaboration with the company's Chemotherapy Research Department in Groton, Connecticut and Agricultural Research Department in Terre Haute. The collaborative invention and discovery of pyrantel included inventors, Lloyd Conover (who also produced the first semisynthetic tetracycline), Bill Austin, and Jim McFarland, along with parasitologists, John Lynch and Harold Howes from Groton, Rendle

Cornwell and Mervyn Jones from Sandwich, and Vasillios Theodorides from Terra Haute. The collaborative medicinal chemistry and drug discovery screening was led by Lloyd Conover in Groton and Bill Austin in Sandwich with some controversy on both sides with the Groton and Sandwich research teams working as competitors to some extent [4].

1.2 DISCOVERY OF PYRANTEL, MORANTEL, AND OXANTEL

During the mid to late 1950s, Pfizer researchers at Groton, Connecticut, established a screening program to find new anthelmintic agents, employing infections of the gastrointestinal nematodes *Nematospiroides dubius* (*Heligmosomoides polygyrus bakeri*) in mice and *Nippostrongylus muris* in rats [5]. In 1959, Lynch and Nelson [6] in Groton modified the *N. dubius* screen of the earlier work of Baker [7] and Hewitt and Gumble [8] by increasing the number of drug doses given prior to evaluation. In their study, mice were infected orally with 40 larvae of *N. dubius* and treated 15 days later with two to five oral doses of the isothiuronium salt, 2-thenylmercapto-2-imidazoline (designated Compound 1871, **6**) (Fig. 1.4) at 12.5−200 mg/kg or in single doses of 12.5−300 mg/kg. All mice were euthanized 2−3 days after termination of the treatment regimen. Appropriate multiple or single doses of the drug were capable of bringing about a greater than 90% reduction in worm burden of the treated mice.

However, while the isothiuronium salt possessed anthelmintic activity against *N. dubius*, it showed little activity when administered orally to sheep, probably due to the high susceptibility of imidazolidines toward rapid metabolism and hydrolysis forming 2-thenylthiol (7) and 2-imidazolidone (8) (Fig. 1.5) [9,10].

While evaluating mouse-derived anthelmintic leads against gastrointestinal nematodes of sheep, a precursor compound of pyrantel containing sulfur in a side chain was tested in Terra Haute. After it was administered to sheep, the barn, environs, field hands, and laboratory personnel became unwittingly exposed to a highly disagreeable odor. The odor was retained

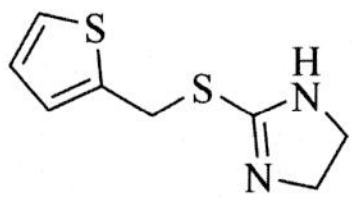

Compound 1871
6

Figure 1.4 Compound 1871 (**6**).

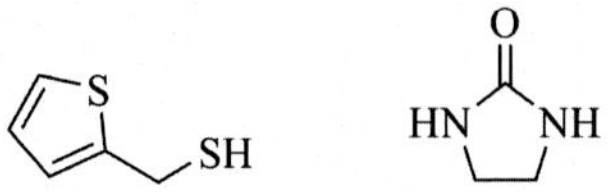

2-Thenylthiol
7

2-Imidazolidone
8

Figure 1.5 Compound 1871 metabolites.

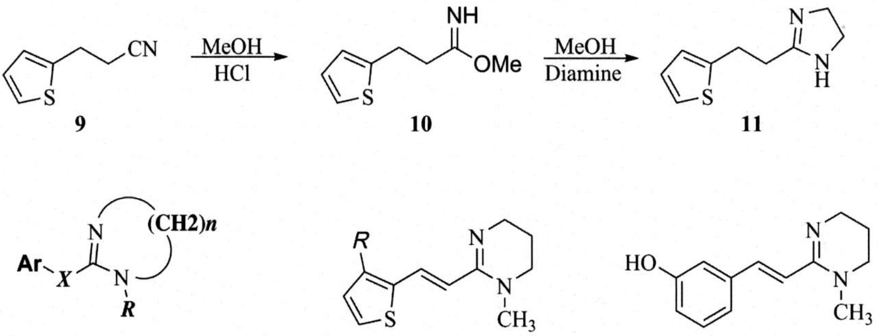

9   **10**   **11**

12   **1** *R*=H   **3**
              2 *R*=Me

Ar=Thienyl, Furyl, Phenyl, etc.
X=Alkyl, Alkenyl
R=Alkyl
n=2 or 3

Figure 1.6 Chemical series leading to synthesis of pyrantel, morantel and oxantel.

on clothing and even the laboratory records of the study. The synthetic chemists at Pfizer were promptly informed that such a product would not be commercially acceptable, regardless of the anthelmintic activity.

The structure of 1871, however, provided a useful lead to follow. New compounds, lacking the aliphatic sulfur (and the disagreeable odor) were prepared. In order to widen the scope of the screens and spectrum of anthelmintic activity, laboratory mice were artificially infected with three distinct parasites. Triple parasite infections in mice included two nematode suborders (Strongylata, Ascaridata) and one cestode order (Cyclophyllidea) that covered three intestinal niches within the host (the duodenum, ileum, and cecum). This screening model was accomplished by acquiring mice with natural infections of *Syphacia obvelata* and *Aspicularis tetraptera*, inoculated with 40 larvae of *N. dubius*, and 5000 ova of *Hymenolepis nana* [11,12].

The discovery of 1871 led to the synthesis of 2[2-(2-thienyl)ethyl]-2-imidazoline (**11**) having activity against different roundworms in mice and sheep [5]. Compound **11** was synthesized by the reaction sequence shown in Fig. 1.6 [13]. Soon a series of compounds of type **12** were prepared of which pyrantel (**1**), morantel (**2**) and oxantel (**3**) showed high anthelmintic activity in the various rodent screening models [14–16]. The compounds of this series are generally prepared by reaction of the imino-ethers derived from the requisite 3-(2-thienyl)propionitrile (**9**), 3-(2-thienyl) acrylonitrile, or their corresponding amides with the appropriate diamine in refluxing methanol or ethanol [15]. Alternatively, in the case of those with a saturated chain, the nitrile may be allowed to react directly with the diamine in the presence of *p*-toluene sulfonic acid (at 175°C), hydrogen sulfide or phosphorus pentasulfide (70–95°C). The final products can be isolated by standard chromatographic procedures.

From this modification effort emerged pyrantel, which, although very active against the mouse helminths, was only moderately active against sheep nematodes. At that time it was customary to dissolve the compounds only in distilled water prior to drenching of the sheep, which severely handicapped the activity of nonaqueous compounds. When it was decided to compare the compound, pyrantel, solubilized in water, or 0.1 N hydrochloric acid, or suspended in aluminum hydroxide gel, a high degree of efficacy was noted in sheep dosed with the acidified compound. A confirmatory experiment was subsequently performed with pyrantel dissolved in 1% tartaric acid solution. The efficacy again was extremely high. This information was transmitted to the chemists, leading to pyrantel tartrate as the preferred salt [10].

1.3 STRUCTURE ACTIVITY RELATIONSHIPS

Following the discovery of pyrantel in 1966, a systematic structure activity relationship (SAR) in compounds of type **12** was carried out to determine the effect of various structural changes on biological activity [12]. Optimal anthelmintic activity in structure **12** was obtained when Ar was 2-thienyl. The structure activity studies revealed that various aryl systems decreased in potency in the order: 2-thienyl > 3-thienyl > phenyl > 2-furyl [14]. Similarly, the presence of a tetrahydropyrimidine ring ($n = 3$) was found to confer better activity as compared to the imidazoline ring ($n = 2$). The presence of a methyl group ($R = Me$) in tetrahydropyrimidine was found essential for evoking high anthelmintic response. It was found that replacement of R by H reduces the activity, while introduction of groups larger than methyl (eg, ethyl, propyl) caused loss of activity. The nature of the linkage (X) joining the 2-thienyl and tetrahydropyrimidine rings in structure **12** also appeared to play an important role in governing the activity. A two carbon chain was required for high activity with the following decreasing order of potency: *trans*-vinylene > ethylene >*cis*-vinylene [5,9]. The following combined structural features appeared to be necessary for optimal anthelmintic activity: (1) a positively charged tail group; (2) a simple aromatic head group; and (3) a two carbon atom chain separating the positive charge from the aromatic ring [17,18] (Fig. 1.7).

It was also observed that in the aromatic head group (Ar = 2-thienyl), the presence of substituents on other positions of the ring, except ortho to linkage, caused loss of activity; morantel (2), having a methyl group at 3-position ("ortho" to vinylene) exhibited a high order of activity. Compounds 1, 2, 13−16 (Fig. 1.8) tested in vivo against *N. dubius* in mice and *Ni. muris* in rats demonstrated anthelmintic activity in roughly that order with pyrantel (1) and morantel (2) being the most active of this series [14].

A quantitative structure activity model was also constructed using the well-known Hansch-Fujita method to derive a multiple linear regression model comprised of two physical descriptors: a measure of the lipophilicity constant (π) for the molecule; and the electron donating coefficient

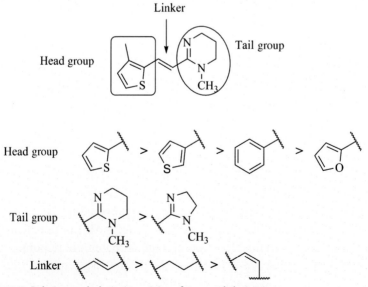

Figure 1.7 Relative anthelmintic activity of pyrantel derivatives.

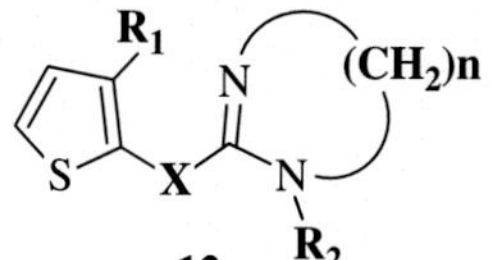

Compound	R_1	R_2	X	n
13	H	H	$-CH_2-CH_2-$	2
14	H	H	$-CH_2-CH_2-$	3
15	H	CH_3	$-CH_2-CH_2-$	2
16	H	CH_3	$-CH_2-CH_2-$	3
1 (Pyrantel)	H	CH_3	$-CH=CH-$	3
2 (Morantel)	CH_3	CH_3	$-CH=CH-$	3

Figure 1.8 Aromatic head group effects on anthelmintic activity.

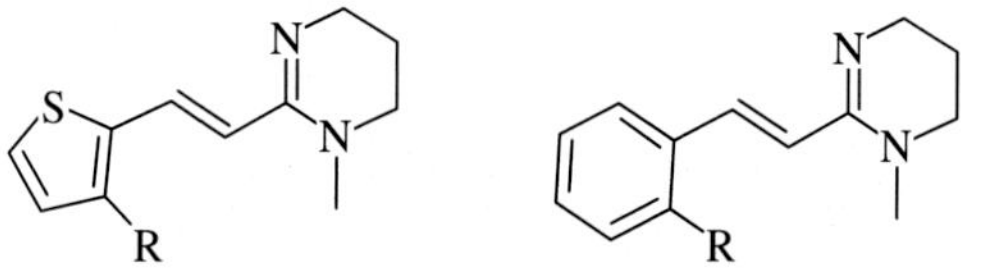

Class A
R = H, Me, Et, Br

Class B
R = H, Cl, Br, F, Me, Et, NO_2

$$Log (1/ED_{90}) = -1.64\pi^2 + 1.93\pi + 0.66\sigma + 0.88$$
$$n = 12, r^2 = 0.962, s = 0.117, F = 84.7, p \leq 0.0005$$

Figure 1.9 Hansch-Fujita analysis and multiple linear regression model of Pyrantel SAR.

of the molecule (σ) [17]. Using this approach, a model was derived that accounted for 96% of the variance of the biological activity for molecules represented by both Class A and Class B (Fig. 1.9) [9].

A number of noncyclic amidines (17), dihydrothiazines and thiazolines (18−20) and 1-(2-arylvinyl) pyridinium salts (21, 22) were also synthesized [13], many of which exhibit marked anthelmintic activity [18−21]. The SAR in many of these series was found to be in close concordance with the tetrahydropyrimidines (Fig. 1.10).

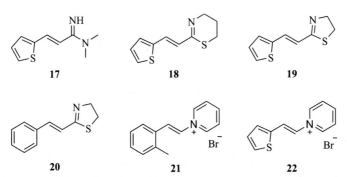

Figure 1.10 Structures of noncyclic amidines (**21**), dihydrothiazines and thiazolines (**18–20**), and 1-(2-arylvinyl pyrimidinium salts (**21, 22**).

1.4 SYNTHESIS OF TETRAHYDROPYRIMIDINE DRUGS

Initially, the cyclic amidines were typically prepared from the requisite 2-arylacrylonitrile (**27**), which is easily obtained by condensation of an aryl aldehyde with cyanoacetic acid followed by decarboxylation. A Pinner reaction involving treatment of **27** with ethanol in the presence of dry HCl, yields ethyl-2-arylacrylimide hydrochloride (**28**), which is condensed with *N*-methyl-1,3-diaminopropane to afford the desired tetrahydropyrimidines, pyrantel (**1**), morantel (**2**), and oxantel (**3**) [13,22−26]. An improved synthesis for preparing **1**, **2** and **3** involves the key intermediate 1,4,5,6-tetrahydro-1,2-dimethylpyrimidine (**26**, R = Me), which may be prepared starting from acrylonitrile (**23**). Addition of an alkyl amine to acrylonitrile affords 2-alkylaminopropionitrile (**24**). Acetylation of the latter with acetic anhydride followed by hydrogenation of the resulting acetyl derivative (**25**) in the presence of Raney nickel catalyst and alcoholic ammonia yields the 1,4,5,6-tetrahydropyrimidines (**26**) [27]. Alternately, the reaction of *N*-methyl-1,3-diaminopropane with an excess of aliphatic nitrile gives 1-methyl-2-alkyl-1,4,5,6-tetrahydropyrimidines (**26**) in the presence of hydrogen sulfide, or a hydrogen sulfide-producing compound, in excellent yields at modest temperature [13] (Fig. 1.11).

A simpler large-scale method to obtain pyrantel, morantel, and oxantel involves condensation of Structure **26** with an aryl aldehyde in the presence of a base. Water is removed by azeotropic distillation or by using an acid dehydrating agent, which scavenges water to push the reaction in the forward direction. Other methods to prepare pyrantel and its derivatives are also reported [12,16,22−26].

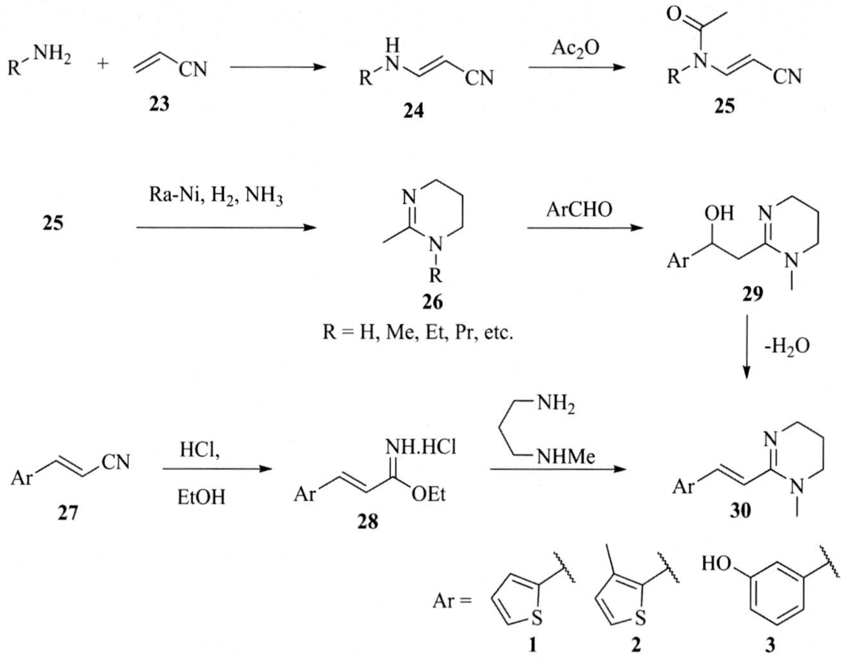

Figure 1.11 Synthesis of Tetrahydropyrimidine drugs.

1.5 PHYSICOCHEMICAL CHARACTERISTICS AND ANTHELMINTIC ACTIVITIES

Pyrantel, morantel, and oxantel emerged as the primary anthelmintics from the discovery campaign, each with their own specific chemical properties and spectra of anthelmintic activities. Various salts of these three compounds were commercialized to meet commercial anthelmintic needs at the time.

1.5.1 Pyrantel and Salts

1.5.1.1 Pyrantel

From the parent Pyrantel (*trans*-1,4,5,6-tetrahydro-1-methyl-2-[2-(2-thienyl) vinyl] pyrimidine), various salts (pamoate, citrate, hydrochloride, and tartrate) have been studied as oral and in-feed anthelmintics for various host species. The anthelmintic activity of the pyrantel salts has been found to be directly proportional to the amount of the free base present. Pyrantel is the most widely used of all the tetrahydropyrimidines anthelmintics. Generally, pyrantel shows high activity against adult nematodes in the lumen of the gastrointestinal tract, but possesses less efficacy against developing forms and poor activity against arrested larvae [28,29]. Based on the anthelmintic activity of administering pyrantel salts orally for treatment of nematode infections, new modes of drug use emerged with superior disease control achieved using pyrantel prophylactically in the feed of swine and horses (Fig. 1.12).

1.5.1.2 Pyrantel Pamoate (Embonate)

Pyrantel is principally available in formulations for dogs and cats as the pamoate (US Pharmacopeia) or embonate (European Pharmacopoeia) salt, which contains 34.7% pyrantel base. It is a combination of pyrantel and pamoic acid. Pyrantel pamoate (embonate) given orally is effective for removal and control of ascarid and hookworm infections in puppies and dogs (adult *Toxocara canis*, *Toxascaris leonina*, *Ancylostoma tubaeforme*, *An. braziliense*, *Uncinaria stenocephala*), cats (adult *Toxocara cati*, *Toxa. leonina*, *An. caninum*, *An. braziliense*, *U. stenocephala*), horses and ponies (adult and immature *Parascaris equorum*, adult *Strongylus vulgaris*, *S. edentatus*, *S. equinus*, Cyathostomes (*Triodontophorus* spp., *Cyathostomum* spp., *Cylicodontophorus* spp., *Cylicocyclus* spp., *Cylicostephanus* spp., *Poteriostomum* spp.), *Oxyuris equi*, *Anoplocephala perfoliata*), swine (adult *Ascaris suum*, *Oesophagostomum dentatum*), and humans (adult *A. lumbricoides*, *Enterobius vermicularis*, *An. duodenale*, *Necator americanus*). Pyrantel pamoate (embonate) has low aqueous solubility and low systemic availability, which increases the margin of safety and efficacy against gut parasites of pigs, horses, pets, and even humans (Fig. 1.13).

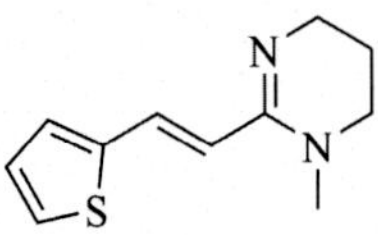

Pyrantel
1

Figure 1.12 Pyrantel (**1**).

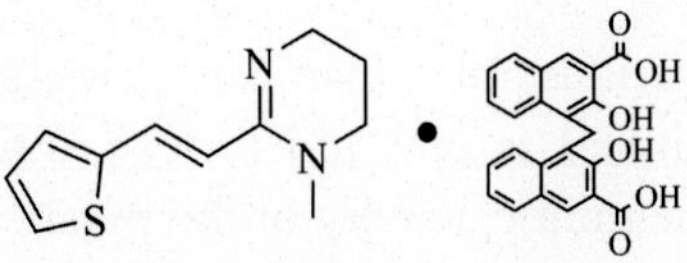

Pyrantel pamoate (embonate)
1a

Figure 1.13 Pyrantel pamoate (**1a**).

1.5.1.3 Pyrantel Citrate

The citrate salt contains 52% pyrantel base. The pharmacokinetics of pyrantel citrate in swine after oral administration showed a mean bio-availability of 41% compared to 16% with pyrantel pamoate [30]. The poor efficacy of pyrantel citrate against nematodes inhabiting the large intestine of pigs was therefore suggested to result from insufficient quantities of the drug passaging to the site of infection. When tested against pyrantel-resistant adult *Oe. dentatum* the efficacy of pyrantel citrate was only 23%, whereas the efficacy of the lesser absorbed pyrantel pamoate was 75%. These results indicate that for maximum activity pyrantel should be administered orally, as opposed to in-feed, to pigs as the pamoate salt. Pyrantel citrate was reported in a laboratory study to be equally effective based on fecal egg count reduction (FECR) and nematode counts (100% at 510 mg of free base/kg of feed) as pyrantel tartrate against *Oe. dentatum* in swine, but in a field study the FECR was 89.4% [31] (Fig. 1.14).

1.5.1.4 Pyrantel Hydrochloride

The hydrochloride salt, contains 85% pyrantel base and is effective in the removal and control of nematode infections in dogs (*Toxo. canis, An. caninum* [32]), swine (*A. suum, Oesophagostomum* spp., *Strongyloides ransomi* [33−35]), and sheep (*Haemonchus contortus, Bunostomum trigonocephalum* and *Ostertagia* spp., *Trichostrongylus* sp., *Oe. venulosum* and *Chabertia ovina* [36]) (Fig. 1.15).

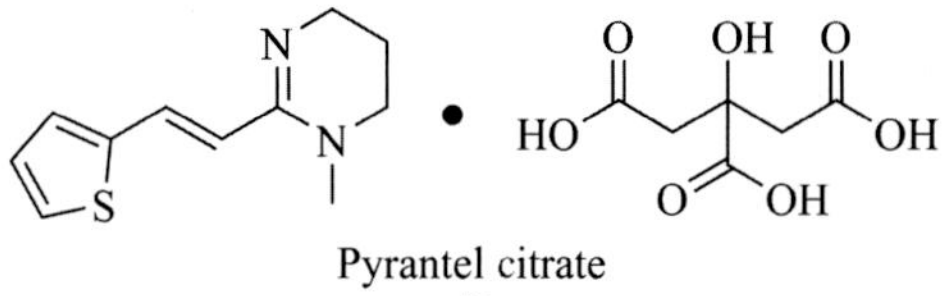

Pyrantel citrate
1b

Figure 1.14 Pyrantel citrate (**1b**).

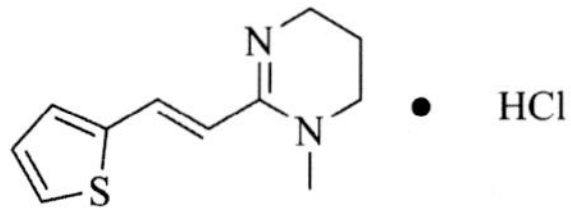

Pyrantel hydrochloride
1c

Figure 1.15 Pyrantel hydrochloride (**1c**).

1.5.1.5 Pyrantel Tartrate

The tartrate salt contains 57.8% pyrantel base. Pyrantel tartrate was particularly active in the triple parasite screen, but had no cestodes activity [11]. In a *Trichinella spiralis* mouse model, pyrantel tartrate in a prophylactic agent test against enteral stages was 81.6% at 50 mg/kg orally. Feed studies of pyrantel tartrate at 0.1% showed 96.7% for 3-day or 95.7% for 6-day schedules, while at 0.5% the tartrate salts showed greater than 98% reduction [11]. Studies in dogs naturally infected with *Taenia pisiformis*, *Dipylidium caninum*, *An. caninum*, *Toxo. canis*, and *Trichuris vulpis* representing the same suborders (Cyclophyllidea, Strongylata, Ascaridata, and Trichurata) as mouse test models showed that a single oral dose of 2.5−25 mg/kg reduced ascarids and hookworm counts greater than 95%, but *Trichu. vulpis* ova counts and worm burdens were not significantly reduced. The spectrum of activity defined by the mouse studies was confirmed in dogs [11]. The therapeutic index of the tartrate salt of pyrantel in sheep is about 7, the broad spectrum minimum effective dose being 25 mg/kg, and the maximum tolerated dose 175 mg/kg [14].

Pyrantel tartrate is an effective drug for treating intestinal roundworm infections in cattle (adult *Ostertagia*, *Trichostrongylus*, *Nematodirus*, *Cooperia* and *Chabertia* spp. [37]), sheep (adult *Nem. battus*, *Ha. contortus*, *Tric. colubriformis* [38,39]), goats (adult *Ha. contortus*, *Teladorsagia circumcincta*, *Tric. colubriformis* [40]), horses (adult *S. vulgaris*, *S. edentatus*, small strongyles: *Cyathostomum* spp., *Cylicocyclus* spp., *Cylicostephanus* spp., *Cylicodontophorus* spp., *Poteriostomum* spp., *Triodontophorus* spp., *P. equorum*, *O. equi* [41,42]), and pigs (adult and immature *A. suum*, adult *Hyostrongylus rubidus* and *Oesophagostomum* spp. [43,44]) (Fig. 1.16).

1.5.2 Morantel

Morantel is used mainly in the form of its salts: tartrate, fumarate, citrate, etc. The pharmacokinetics of each salt is slightly different. It is excreted mainly in the feces in the form of the unchanged parent compound.

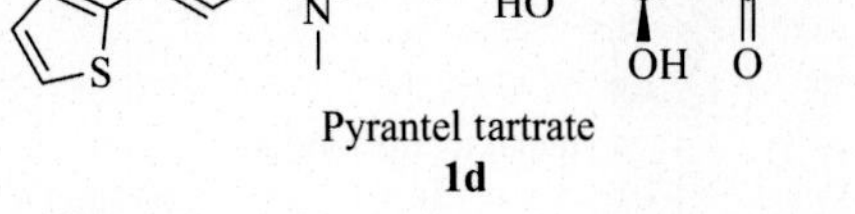

Pyrantel tartrate
1d

Figure 1.16 Pyrantel tartrate (**1d**).

Absorbed morantel is quickly metabolized in the liver. After oral administration to cattle and goats (10 mg/kg) morantel cannot be detected in plasma (<0.05 mcg/mL). In lactating goats, morantel is not detectable in the milk. Four days after oral administration, approximately 17% of the dose is excreted in the urine as polar metabolites, and greater than 70% in the feces as unchanged parent molecule. The activity profile of this drug is almost similar to that of pyrantel except its lower therapeutic dose and higher LD_{50} values. Like pyrantel, the activity of morantel against adult gut nematodes is highest (>90%), less against developing forms (75−90%), and minimal (<50%) against arrested larvae [28].

Morantel has also been found to be highly effective against immature and mature forms of *A. suum* in pigs at a dose of 5 mg/kg. In addition, the drug eliminates adult worms of *Oesophagostomum* and *Hyostrongylus* spp. [28,45]. The uses of morantel in the treatment/prophylaxis of gastrointestinal nematodes in cattle, sheep, horses and dogs has been reviewed [9] (Fig. 1.17).

1.5.2.1 Morantel Citrate

The citrate salt contains 53% morantel base. Morantel citrate is effective against gastrointestinal parasites of sheep (adult *Ha. contortus*, *Trichostrongylus* spp., *Te. circumcincta*, *Tric. axei*, *Cooperia curticei*, *Nematodirus* spp., *Ch. ovina*, *Oe. venulosum* [46]) and swine (adult *A. suum*, *Oe. dentatum*) (Fig. 1.18).

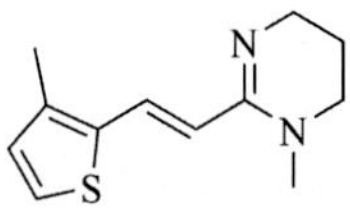

Morantel
2

Figure 1.17 Morantel (**2**).

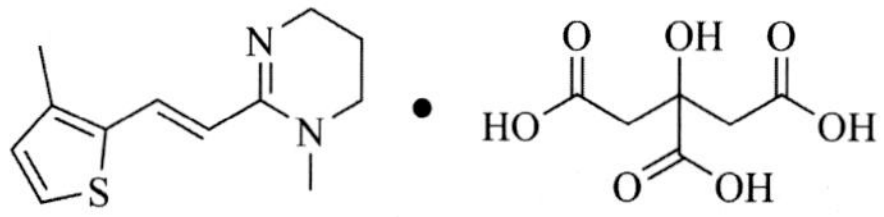

Morantel citrate
2a

Figure 1.18 Morantel citrate (**2a**).

1.5.2.2 Morantel Tartrate

The tartrate salt contains 59% morantel base. After oral administration to ruminants morantel tartrate is very poorly absorbed into the bloodstream. The recommended oral dose of morantel tartrate is 10 mg/kg in medicated feed for treating gastrointestinal nematode infections in cattle (adult *Haemonchus*, *Ostertagia*, *Trichostrongylus*, *Cooperia* spp., *Nematodirus* spp., *Oe. radiatum*) and sheep (adult *Ha. contortus*, *Te. circumcincta*, *Tric. axei*) [28,29,47]. Morantel tartrate for swine in medicated feed at (1250 mg/kg in complete feed) is effective against mature *Hy. rubidus*, mature and immature *A. suum*, and mature and immature *Oesophagostomum* spp. As a paste or oral granule formulation, morantel tartrate is effective against equine gastrointestinal parasites (*Strongylus* spp., Cyathostomes (lumen dwelling immature forms of *Cyathostomum* spp., *Triodontophorus* spp. and *S. vulgaris*), *P. equorum*, *O. equi*, *Ano. perfoliata*) [48,49].

Morantel tartrate was developed as various boluses (Nematel, Paratect Cartridge, and Paratect Flex Diffuser) representing both a revolutionary mode of control of internal worms in grazing cattle and a novel prolonged-release delivery system. The disease-control concept, originated by parasitologists Rendle Cornwell and Mervyn Jones in Sandwich, was based upon their knowledge of the annual parasite life cycle. Continuous release of drug in the first stomach (rumen) of calves for 60–90 days in the spring blocked the parasite "multiplication" stages, and this prevented the harmful infection which naturally occurred in late summer.

The Nematel Cattle Wormer Bolus was effective for the removal and control of species of *Haemonchus*, *Ostertagia*, *Trichostrongylus*, *Cooperia*, *Nematodirus*, and *Oesophagostomum*. The work on improving the drug delivery system continued and produced another new design featuring a drug-infused, perforated-sheet matrix, which was administered in cylindrical form and then was held in the rumen as a flattened sheet.

The Paratect Cartridge bolus consisted of a metal cylinder enclosed at each end by a drug-releasing membrane and was effective for removal and control of *Ostertagia* spp., *Tric. axei*, *Cooperia* spp., and *Oe. radiatum* for approximately 90 days following administration.

The work on improving the drug delivery system continued and produced another new design featuring a drug-infused, perforated-sheet matrix which was administered in cylindrical form, then was held in the rumen as a flattened sheet, Paratect Flex Diffuser [50]. Both in vitro and in vivo release performance of devices containing morantel tartrate were

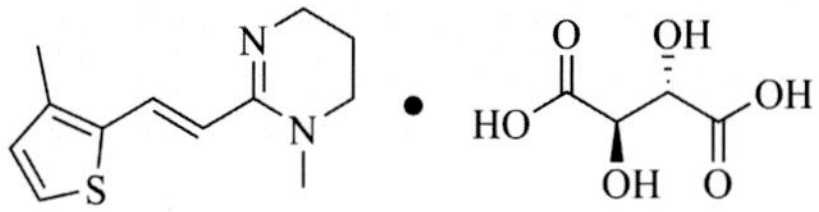

Morantel tartrate
2b

Figure 1.19 Morantel tartrate (**2b**).

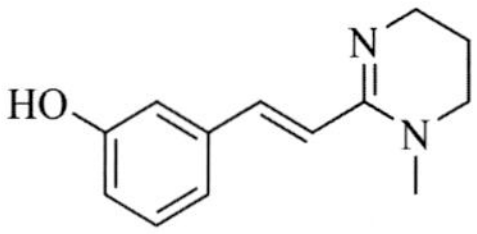

Oxantel
3

Figure 1.20 Oxantel (**3**).

found to compare favorably with one another and demonstrated controlled delivery of morantel for 90 days both in vitro and in vivo. The bolus provided removal and control of *Ostertagia* spp., *Tric. axei*, *Cooperia* spp., and *Oe. radiatum* (Fig. 1.19).

1.5.3 Oxantel

Oxantel is the *m*-oxyphenol analog of pyrantel with particular anthelmintic activity against *Trichuris* spp. It was discovered in the early 1970s by Pfizer and showed high activity in *Trichu. muris*-infected mice and *Trichu. vulpis*-infected dogs [21,51]. This activity against whipworm infection compensated for its narrow spectrum of anthelmintic activity, and became the principal clinical application [52]. Oxantel and its salts in combination with pyrantel pamoate and benzimidiazoles are currently used for the treatment of ascariasis, enterobiasis, hookworm infections, and trichuriasis in humans. Oxantel and pyrantel have been recently combined with praziquantel as a broad-spectrum anthelmintic for dogs to treat *Trichu. vulpis* (99.3% and 100% in experimental and naturally infected dogs, respectively), *Toxo. canis* (94.3% and 100% in experimental and naturally infected dogs, respectively), *An. caninum* (99% fecal egg count reduction), *D. caninum* (proglottids in feces 100%), and *Echinococcus granulosus* (99.9% in experimentally infected dogs) [53] (Fig. 1.20).

1.5.3.1 Oxantel Pamoate (Embonate)

Oxantel is most frequently encountered as the embonate salt, which contains 35.8% oxantel base. Oxantel embonate has low aqueous solubility

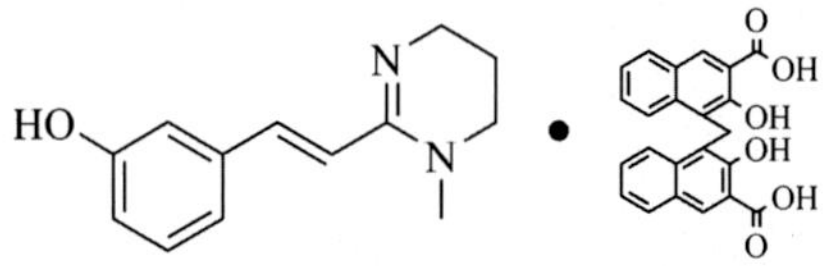

Oxantel pamoate (embonate)
3a

Figure 1.21 Oxantel pamoate (**3a**).

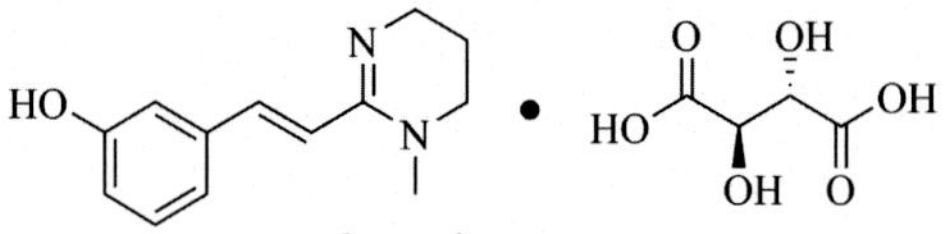

Oxantel tartrate
3b

Figure 1.22 Oxantel tartrate (**3b**).

and little (around 8−10%) is absorbed, permitting the drug to reach high concentrations in the lower gastrointestinal tract sufficient to be effective against whipworms [21]. This drug is particularly useful in treating mild to severe infections of the whipworm *Trichu. trichura*. Oxantel is an extremely well tolerated drug with no severe toxic manifestations. A combination of pyrantel and oxantel exhibited high activity against ascarids, hookworms, and whipworms in cats and dogs at a dose of 100 mg/animal. However, this product was removed from the market with the introduction of other broad-spectrum anthelmintic combinations (Fig. 1.21).

1.5.3.2 Oxantel Tartrate
Oxantel tartrate has been found to be effective against *Trichu. suis*, but has little activity against other intestinal nematodes in pigs [54] (Fig. 1.22).

1.6 CONCLUSION

It has been approximately 55 years since the discovery of the Tetrahydropyrimidine class of anthelmintics. In spite of the new highly active and broad-spectrum anthelmintics introduced into veterinary and human medicine along with the emerging anthelmintic-resistance to this class, the Tetrahydropyrimidines still provide value and utility individually and in combination in the treatment of nematode infections in animals and humans.

REFERENCES

[1] Pfizer (US) Company History [cited 2015 Nov 19]. Available from: http://www.pfizer.com/about/history/all.

[2] Pfizer (UK) Our History 1949-55 [cited 2010 Nov 25]. Available from: http://www.pfizer.co.uk/sites/PfizerCoUK/AboutUs/History/Pages/PfizerWorldwide.aspx.

[3] Pfizer (UK) Our History 1955-70 [cited 2010 Nov 25]. Available from: http://www.pfizer.co.uk/sites/PfizerCoUK/AboutUs/History/Pages/PfizerHistory1955-1970.aspx.

[4] Tanner O. 25 Years of innovation: the story of Pfizer central research. Lyme, CT: Greenwich Publishing Group, Inc.; 1996.

[5] McFarland JW. In: Bindra JS, Lednicer D, editors. Chronicles of drug discovery, vol. 2. New York, NY: John Wiley & Sons; 1983. p. 87–108.

[6] Lynch JE, Nelson B. Preliminary anthelmintic studies with *Nematospiroides dubius* in mice. J Parasitol 1959;45:659–62.

[7] Baker NF. Trichostrongyloidosis—the mouse as an experimental animal. Proc Am Vet Med Assoc 1954;185.

[8] Hewitt R, Gumble A. Effects of standard anthelmintics on experimental infections with *Nematospiroides dubius* Baylis in laboratory mice. J Parasitol 1957;43:18 (section 2).

[9] McFarland JW. The chemotherapy of intestinal nematodes. Prog Drug Res 1972;16:157–93.

[10] Theodorides VJ. Anthelmintics: from laboratory animals to the target species. In: Gadebusch HH, editor. Chemotherapy of infectious disease. 1976. p. 71–94.

[11] Howes Jr HL, Lynch JE. Anthelmintic studies with pyrantel. I. Therapeutic and prophylactic efficacy against the enteral stages of various helminths in mice and dogs. J Parasitol 1967;53(5):1085–91.

[12] McFarland JW, Conover IH, Howes Jr HL, Lynch JE, Chrisholm DR, Austin WC, et al. Novel agents. II. Pyrantel and other cyclic amidines. J Med Chem 1969;12:1066–79.

[13] Anand N. Tetrahydropyrimidines, Chapter 6. Approaches to design and synthesis of antiparasitic drugs. The Netherlands: Elsevier Science B.V.; 1997. p. 171–80.

[14] Austin WC, Courtney W, Danilewicz JC, Morgan DH, Conover LH, Howes Jr HL, et al. Pyrantel tartrate, a new anthelmintic effective against infections of domestic animals. Nature 1966;212:1273–4.

[15] McFarland JW. In: Bindra JS, Lednicer D, editors. Chronicles of drug discovery, vol. 2. New York, NY: John Wiley & Sons; 1983. p. 87–108.

[16] McFarland JW, Howes Jr HL. Novel anthelmintic agents. 6. Pyrantel analogs with activity against whipworm. J Med Chem 1972;15(4):365–8.

[17] McFarland JW. The chemotherapy of intestinal nematodes. Prog Drug Res 1972;16:157–93.

[18] McFarland JW, Howes Jr HL. Novel anthelmintic agents. 3. 1-(2-arylvinyl)pyridinium salts. J Med Chem 1969;12(6):1079–86.

[19] McFarland JW, Howes Jr HL. Novel anthelmintic agents. IV. Noncyclic amidines related to pyrantel. J Med Chem 1970;13:109–13.

[20] McFarland JW, Howes Jr HL, Conover LH, Lynch JE, Austin WC, Morgan DH. Novel anthelmintic agents. V. Thiazoline and dihydrothiazine analogs of pyrantel. J Med Chem 1970;13:113–19.

[21] Howes Jr HL. Trans-1,4,5,6-tetrahydro-2-(3-hydroxystyryl)-1-methyl pyrimidine (CP-14,445), a new antiwhipworm agent. Proc Soc Exp Biol Med 1972;139 (2):394–8.

[22] Pfizer Corp. Belgium Patent 658,987: Chem. Abstr. 1966; 64:8192.

[23] Austin WC, Conover LH, Courtney W, McFarland JW. British Patent 1,120,587: Chem. Abstr. 1968; 68:96768e.

[24] Conover LH, McFarland JW, Austin WCUS. Patent 3,644,624: Chem. Abstr. 1972; 77:5508w.

[25] Kasubick R.V., McFarland J.W. South African Patent 6,800,516: Chem. Abstr. 1969; 70:68406n.

[26] Lelean PM, Morris JA. JCS Chem Commun 1968;239.

[27] Mikolajewska H, Kotelko A. Studies on the hydrogenation of aminonitriles. 8. Catalytic hydrogenation of N-alkyl-N-(2-cyanoethyl)-acetamides. Acta Polen Pharm 1965;22(3):219–24.

[28] Marriner S, Armour J. In: Campbell WC, Rew RS, editors. Chemotherapy of parasitic disease. New York, NY: Plenum Press; 1986. p. 287–305.

[29] Bogan J, Armour J. Anthelmintics for ruminants. Int J Parasitol 1987;17:483–4.

[30] Bjørn H, Hennessy DR, Friis C. The kinetic disposition of pyrantel citrate and pamoate and their efficacy against pyrantel-resistant Oesphogastomum in pigs. Int J Parasitol 1996;26(12):1375–80.

[31] Pratt SE, Brauer MA, Corwin RM. Relative efficacies of pyrantel tartrate and pyrantel citrate against Oesophagostomum sp in swine. Am J Vet Res 1981;42(5):871–2.

[32] Bradley RE, Conway DP. Evaluation of pyrantel hydrochloride as an anthelmintic in dogs. Vet Med Small Anim Clin 1970;65(8):767–9.

[33] Zimmermann DR, Speer VC, Zimmermann W, Switzer WP. Effect of pyrantel salts on Ascaris suum infections in growing pigs. J Anim Sci 1971;32:874–8.

[34] Forrester DJ, Handlin DL, Skelley GC. Pyrantel hydrochloride as an anthelmintic agent against Ascaris suum and Oesophagostomum spp. in swine. Technical Bulletin, South Carolina Agricultural Experiment Station, Clemson University; 1970. pp. (i)+13 pp.

[35] Hale O, Stewart TB, Johnson JC. Response of parasitized pigs to pyrantel HCl and dietary protein. J Anim Sci 1971;33(1):231.

[36] Danek J, Sevcrik B. Efficacy of various pyrantel salts in a critical test in sheep. [Czech.]. Veterinaria, Sofa 1972;14(2):91–102.

[37] Cornwell RL, Jones RM. Controlled laboratory trials with pyrantel tartrate in cattle 1970 Brit Vet J 1970;126(3):134–41.

[38] Cornwell RL, Berry J, Light TC, Mercer EA, Phillips G. Field trials in sheep with the anthelmintic pyrantel tartrate. I. Comparative trials in the prevention of Nematodirus infection in lambs. Vet Rec 1966;79(22):626–9.

[39] Cornwell RL. Controlled laboratory trials in sheep with the anthelmintic pyrantel tartrate. Vet Rec 1966;79(21):590–5.

[40] Chartier C, Pors I, Benoit C. Efficacy of pyrantel tartrate against experimental infections with Haemonchus contortus, Teladorsagia circumcincta and Trichostrongylus colubriformis in goats. Vet Parasitol 1995;59(1):69–73.

[41] Conway DP, DeGoosh C, Chalquest RR. Clinical studies of the anthelmintic pyrantel tartrate in horses. Vet Med Small Anim Clin 1970;65(9):899 passim.

[42] Lyons ET, Drudge JH, Tolliver SC, Breukink HJ. Critical tests of three salts of pyrantel against internal parasites of the horse. Am J Vet Res 1974;35(2):1515–22.

[43] Wescott RB, Walker JH. Efficacy of pyrantel tartrate as an anthelmintic in swine. Am J Vet Res 1970;31(3):567–9.

[44] Kennedy TJ, Conway DP, Bliss DH. Prophylactic medication with pyrantel to prevent liver condemnation in pigs naturally exposed to Ascaris infections. Am J Vet Res 1980;41(12):2089–91.

[45] Raether W. In: Melhorn H, editor. Parasitology in focus: facts and trends. Heidelberg: Springer Verlag; 1988. p. 739–866.

[46] Austin WC, Cornwell RL, Jones RM. Anthelmintic activity in sheep of some compounds related to pyrantel and morantel. J Med Chem 1972;15(3):281–5.

[47] Johnson CK, Pinkston ML. Controlling endoparasites in dairy cattle with morantel tartrate. Vet Med 1988;83(10):1074–7.

[48] Cornwell RL, Jones RM, Pott JM. Critical trials of morantel tartrate in equine strongylosis. Vet Rec 1973;93(4):94—8.

[49] Cornwell RL, Jones RM, Pott JM. Critical trials with morantel tartrate against *Parascaris equorum*. Res Vet Sci 1973;14(1):134—6.

[50] Boettner WA, Aguiar AJ, Cardinal JR, Curtiss AC, Ranade GR, Richards JA, et al. The morantel sustained release trilaminate: a device for the controlled ruminal delivery of morantel to cattle. J Control Release 1988;8(1):23—30.

[51] Rajasekariah GR, Deb BN, Jones MP, Dhage KR, Bose S. Response of pre-adult and adult stages of *Trichuris muris* to common anthelmintics in mice. Int J Parasitol 1991;21:697—702.

[52] Lee EL, Iyngkaran N, Greive AW, Robinson MJ, Dissanaike AS. Therapeutic evaluation of oxantel pamoate (1,4,5,6-tetrahydro-1-methyl-2-[trans-3-hydroxystyryl] pyrimidine pamoate) in severe *Trichuris trichura* infection 1979 Am J Trop Med Hyg 1979;25:563—7.

[53] Schmid K, Rohdich N, Zschiesche E, Kok DJ, Allan MJ. Efficacy, safety and palatability of a new broad-spectrum anthelmintic formulation in dogs. Vet Rec 2010;167(17):647—51.

[54] Robinson M. Efficacy of oxantel tartrate against *Trichuris suis* in swine. Vet Parasitol 1979;5(2—3):223—35.

CHAPTER 2

Pharmacology of Pyrantel

R.J. Martin[1] and T.G. Geary[2]
[1]Department of Biomedical Sciences, College of Veterinary Medicine, Iowa State University, Ames, IA, United States
[2]Institute of Parasitology, McGill University, St. Anne de Bellevue, QC, Canada

2.1 INTRODUCTION

Pyrantel and its analogs (oxantel and morantel) are members of the tetrahydropyrimidine family that were developed by Pfizer in the 1960s and marketed from the 1970s as veterinary anthelmintics; they were subsequently adapted for use in human medicine. Pyrantel is sometimes described as a narrow spectrum anthelmintic, but this is the case when compared to the macrocyclic lactone endectocides, which have spectra that extend beyond gastrointestinal (GI) parasitic nematodes to include lung-worm, filariae, and even some arthropods. Pyrantel has significant efficacy against a fairly wide range of GI nematodes and remains of considerable therapeutic value. The main features of its mode of action are now understood, while mechanisms of resistance to pyrantel are beginning to be unraveled. In this chapter, we review the properties of pyrantel, consider aspects of its mode of action and pharmacology, and comment on resistance.

2.2 PHARMACOLOGY

2.2.1 Pyrantel Structure and Discovery

In 1966, a publication in *Nature* entitled, "A new series of highly active anthelmintic compounds which exhibit a broad spectrum of activity against both adult and immature worm infections of domestic animals," announced the discovery of pyrantel and its analogs [1]. That series is shown in Fig. 2.1, modified from the original publication to show the structures of pyrantel (V) and morantel (IV). The anthelmintic activity of these compounds was discovered in screens employing infections of the GI parasites *Nematospiroides dubius* (*Heligmosomoides polygyrus bakeri*) in mice and *Nippostrongylus muris* in rats. Compound V, which became known as pyrantel, was reported to be effective at a dose of 25 mg/kg

Pyrantel Parasiticide Therapy in Humans and Domestic Animals.
DOI: http://dx.doi.org/10.1016/B978-0-12-801449-3.00013-2
21

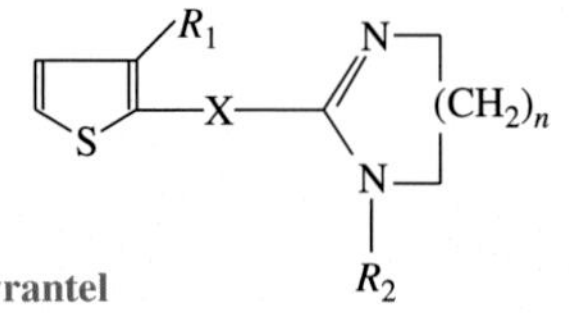

V = pyrantel

(I) R_1 = H R_2 = H X = $-CH_2CH_2-$ n = 2

(II) R_1 = H R_2 = H X = $-CH_2CH_2-$ n = 3

(III) R_1 = H R_2 = CH_3 X = $-CH_2CH_2-$ n = 2

(IV) R_1 = H R_2 = CH_3 X = $-CH_2CH_2-$ n = 3

(V) R_1 = H R_2 = CH_3 X = $-CH=CH_2-$ n = 3

(VI) R_1 = CH_3 R_2 = CH_3 X = $-CH=CH_2-$ n = 3

Figure 2.1 Chemical structures, including pyrantel (blue) and morantel (red), developed and tested by Pfizer. *From Austin W, Courtney W, Danilewi JC, Morgan D, Conover L, Howes H, et al. Pyrantel tartrate, a new anthelmintic effective against infections of domestic animals. Nature 1966;212(5067):1273–4.*

Oxantel

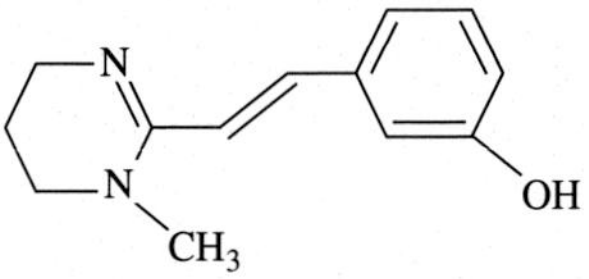

Figure 2.2 Chemical structure of oxantel.

against adult and immature *Haemonchus*, *Ostertagia*, *Trichostrongylus*, *Nematodirus*, *Cooperia*, and *Trichostrongylus* species in cattle and sheep. The therapeutic index of the tartrate salt of pyrantel was reported to be about 7. Interestingly, doses that were safe and therapeutic for other nematodes were, for as yet unclear reasons, found to have limited efficacy against species in the genus *Trichuris* (whipworms). The limited efficacy of pyrantel against *Trichuris* species was recognized early on and, as a result, oxantel (Fig. 2.2) was developed for the treatment of *Trichuris* and is especially employed for this indication in pigs [2].

Pyrantel is defined in the US Pharmacopeia as having the formula $C_{11}H_{14}N_2S$, with a molecular weight of 206 D and the IUPAC name 4-[(3-carboxy-2-hydroxynaphthalen-1-yl)methyl]-3-hydroxynaphthalene-2-carboxylic acid; 1-methyl-2-[(E)-2-thiophen-2-ylethenyl]-5,6-dihydro-4H-pyrimidine. It is usually used as the pamoate/embonate salt: pamoate is the US Pharmacopeia name, and the embonate is the European name. The pamoate/embonate salt has a molecular composition of $C_{23}H_{16}O_6$ with a molecular weight of 389 D. The USP pyrantel pamoate preparation contains not less than 97% of the salt. Pyrantel is also available as the tartrate or citrate salts, which are considerably more soluble and bioavailable preparations.

2.2.2 Therapeutic Actions Against GI Nematodes

Pyrantel pamoate (Strongid, Nemocid) may be used for the treatment of hookworms and roundworms in humans, pets, and other animals with effects that can vary according to parasite species and resistance status [3]. Hookworms and *Trichuris* species are typically less susceptible to pyrantel than *Ascaris* species and related roundworms [3]. Pyrantel is most commonly used in pigs for *Ascaris suum* and *Oesophagostomum dentatum*, in horses for ascarids, large and small strongyles and oxyurids (and at a double dose for *Anoplocephala*), and as a broad spectrum GI anthelmintic in ruminants. In dogs and cats, pyrantel is used for common GI nematodes, except whipworms. In humans, it is used to treat pinworms, round-worms, and hookworms [4]. For pinworms, the medication may be used for self-treatment, but for other infections, medical advice is desirable and treatment of children less than 2 years old should be avoided.

Oxantel pamoate (Fig. 2.2) is primarily used for the treatment of whipworms (*Trichuris*), an indication for which pyrantel is largely ineffective. Part of the reason oxantel is effective against whipworms is that this drug is poorly absorbed from the GI tract and reaches a higher concentration in the large intestine where whipworms are found. Thus, part of the reason for its efficacy against whipworms is its pharmacokinetic properties; another reason may relate to different nicotinic receptor subtypes present in whipworms.

Interestingly, oxantel, in addition to its other cholinergic effects, is an inhibitor of fumarate reductase and reduces the ability of oral bacteria to produce chronic periodontitis [5]. As a result of its inhibitory effects on spirochetes, it has been advocated for dental use.

Morantel (Rumatel) is structurally closely related to pyrantel: it is the 3-methyl thiophene analog of pyrantel and has been used in ruminants as the tartrate salt since 1981. It is commercially available in four formulations: medicated premix, cattle wormer bolus, oral suspension, and sustained release bolus. It is not licensed for human use. It is effective against upper GI nematodes such as *Haemonchus*, *Ostertagia*, and *Trichostrongylus* species in cattle [3].

2.3 MECHANISM OF ACTION

2.3.1 Molecular and Cellular Mechanisms

Fig. 2.3 reproduces part of the original figures published on the mechanism of action of pyrantel [6]. That manuscript illustrates many of the salient features of the mechanism of pyrantel action. Fig. 2.3a shows that

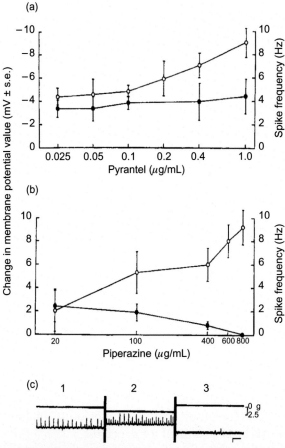

Figure 2.3 The pharmacological effects of pyrantel on *A. suum* body muscle. (a) Concentration-dependent effects of pyrantel and (b) piperazine on spike frequency (excitation) and membrane potential. (c) Effects of pyrantel and piperazine on membrane potential and contraction; the top trace shows contraction and the lower trace intracellular membrane potential; 1 is the control recording, 2 is the effect of pyrantel showing contraction and depolarization and increased spiking, 3 is the effect of adding piperazine (9 mM) on top of pyrantel producing hyperpolarization and relaxations and countering the effect of pyrantel (1.1 μM). *From Austin W, Courtney W, Danilewi JC, Morgan D, Conover L, Howes H, et al. Pyrantel tartrate, a new anthelmintic effective against infections of domestic animals. Nature 1966;212(5067):1273−4.*

pyrantel has depolarizing and excitatory effects on muscle membrane in *Ascaris* muscle preparations. Concentrations greater than or equal to 0.2 μg/mL (0.56 μM pyrantel tartrate) produce depolarization and increase spike frequency. In Fig. 2.3c, the lowest trace (compare 1 to 2) shows that 0.4 μg/mL pyrantel (1.1 μM pyrantel tartrate) produces a depolarization of 6 mV (-34 to -28 mV) and an increase in spike frequency (3.7–4.1 Hz). The bottom trace in Fig. 2.3c (compare 2 to 3) shows that adding 7.7 mM piperazine to pyrantel hyperpolarizes the membrane potential to -38 mV and abolishes spike activity, completely reversing the effect of pyrantel. The top trace in Fig. 2.3c (compare 1 to 2) shows that the application of pyrantel contracts the preparation, and the addition of piperazine (compare 2 to 3) counters the effect of pyrantel and produces relaxation. The effects of pyrantel were also antagonized by *d*-tubocurarine, a well-characterized nicotinic cholinergic antagonist, emphasizing the nicotinic nature of the receptor activated by pyrantel. Interestingly, the authors of this early paper did not explicitly state that pyrantel is a selective nematode nAChR agonist, but say something close: "…effects on preparations of *Ascaris* in which pyrantel and its analogues showed marked persistent nicotinic properties resulted in spastic paralysis of the worm." These authors clearly understood the basic mechanism of action of pyrantel, but did not investigate the reasons for differences in sensitivity of nAChRs of parasitic nematodes and their hosts.

We now understand more about the mechanism of action of pyrantel, which clearly is a nicotinic acetylcholine receptor (nAChR) agonist. The endogenous ligand for these receptors, acetylcholine (ACh), can activate two main types of receptor: ionotropic receptors (nAChR channels composed of five transmembrane subunits that surround and form a cation-permeable pore); and metabotropic receptors, typically termed muscarinic ACh receptors (seven-transmembrane receptors coupled to αβγ G-proteins). Pyrantel activates ionotropic receptors as an agonist like ACh (Fig. 2.4) but lacks activity against muscarinic receptors.

2.3.2 Ionotropic Receptors of Pyrantel, nAChRs

Pyrantel mimics the effects of ACh as an agonist, but only binds with high affinity to a subtype of nematode nAChRs. The pyrantel-sensitive subtypes of nAChRs are likely to be made up of subunits named UNC-63, UNC-38, UNC-29 (two of these), and ACR-8 [7,8]. Following binding of the agonist, the channel opens and allows the cations: Na^+, K^+, and Ca^{2+} to

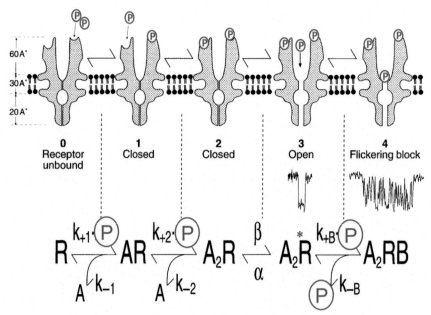

Figure 2.4 Diagram of a nAChR channel in the membrane (top) and the binding of two agonist (pyrantel) molecules to the canonical ligand binding sites (usually two) in steps (0−1−2) that are separated kinetically and which lead, after binding of two molecules, to a brief opening [3] of the channel that lasts around 1 ms and allows a current of 1.5 pA to enter the cell through the membrane. The channel may then close or a third molecule of agonist may enter the open channel and oscillate in and out of the open-channel pore to produce a flickering channel block [4]. A kinetic diagram and rate constants governing the agonist and channel block action are shown (bottom).

move through the channel [8]. Agonists such as pyrantel bind to sites on the assembled receptor which are located between two of the subunits; one side of a binding site (the principle site) is formed by alpha–subunits (UNC-63, UNC-38, or ACR-8) that have two vicinal cysteine residues, and the other side (the complementary site) is formed by a non–alpha subunit (UNC-29). Fig. 2.4 shows a diagrammatic representation of the sequential binding of two pyrantel molecules (P) to open the channel and a kinetic diagram, in which the agonist (A: pyrantel) binds to two sites to produce the opening of the channel (*). Fig. 2.4 also shows how pyrantel, which is a cation, can enter the open channel and produce a flickering open–channel block of the channel [9]. Pyrantel is a potent nAChR agonist and can open this subtype of nAChRs at concentrations greater than or equal to 0.1 μM, and can produce open–channel block with a dissociation constant of 20 μM at −75 mV [9]. Thus, the agonist effect, rather than the open channel block, predominates in parasitic nematodes at therapeutic doses. In contrast, the dissociation constant of pyrantel for channel block at vertebrate nAChRs is similar (8 μM at −75 mV), but the drug acts as a low efficacy agonist [10]. It is interesting that pyrantel acts both as an agonist and an antagonist in both parasites and their hosts, but it is the agonist action that is the primary source of therapeutic selectivity.

It is thus clear that pyrantel is a potent nAChR agonist, but the molecular bases for host−parasite selectivity in the potency of pyrantel are only recently becoming evident. As noted, pyrantel is a potent agonist of nematode muscle nAChRs, but only a partial agonist on some mammalian muscle nAChRs. A partial explanation of this difference was obtained from mutation studies [11], which illustrated the role of individual amino acids at the binding site on the complementary face (the non-alpha subunit). The amino acid at position 57 on the complementary face of the binding site was shown to play a key role in the selective activation of nAChRs by pyrantel. The presence of glycine at position 57 in the mammalian muscle nAChR causes pyrantel to behave as a partial agonist. In contrast, when glutamine occupies position 57, as in the nematode muscle nAChR, pyrantel behaves as a full agonist. The early studies of Aubry et al. [6] reported that pyrantel has cholinergic partial agonist (and sometimes antagonist) effects on vertebrate preparations. Interestingly, pyrantel increases cat blood pressure when injected intravenously, revealing a ganglionic nAChR agonist effect, and causes spastic paralysis when injected in chick veins, showing an agonist action on avian nAChRs. Subsequent studies [12,13] reported the allosteric effects of pyrantel, morantel, and oxantel on vertebrate neuronal nAChRs (α3β2 and α4β2) expressed in *Xenopus* oocytes. Morantel and pyrantel potentiates the opening of α3β2 receptors, but oxantel inhibits the opening of α4β2. Thus, these compounds have the potential to interact in different ways with various mammalian nAChR subtypes, depending on their subunit structure, and are therapeutically safer if they are restricted to the GI tract by using the embonate/pamoate rather than the tartrate or citrate salt.

2.3.3 Patch-Clamp Recordings

Pyrantel-induced changes in the opening and closing of nAChRs can be observed with the patch-clamp recording technique, in which a fire-polished micropipette containing pyrantel is placed over nAChRs present in the muscle membrane in a nematode tissue preparation, as illustrated for *O. dentatum* (Fig. 2.5a). The nematodes are firstly micro–dissected (Fig. 2.5b) and then treated with collagenase to clean muscle membranes and produce vesicles (Fig. 2.5c) suitable for patch–clamp recording. A patch–pipette containing pyrantel is then placed on the surface of the muscle cell and the current flowing up the pipette is recorded as the channel opens and closes under the influence of pyrantel.

The opening and closing of nAChRs produces rectangular pulses, allowing small currents of about 1 pA to be observed (Fig. 2.5c). The inward current carries Na^+ and Ca^{2+} ions which produce depolarization of the membrane potential and, in intact muscle cells, consequent contraction. Characterization of the properties of single–channel currents in muscle preparations from *O. dentatum* has revealed some unexpected properties of these nAChRs and their activation by cholinergic anthelmintics, including pyrantel.

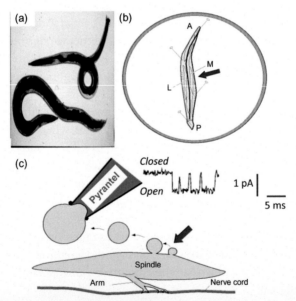

Figure 2.5 (a) Photograph of live, unstained, female and male *O. dentatum*. The female is about 1 cm in length and is bigger than the male. (b) Diagram of dissection of a female worm in a Petri-dish under a dissecting microscope. Individual muscle cells can be seen (M); the lateral line (L) separates the dorsal and ventral halves of the worm. (c) Exposure of the flap preparation to a brief application of collagenase to erode the extracellular matrix leads to the production of micro-vesicles that are suitable for patch-clamp recording of single channel currents activated by pyrantel.

The relationship between the amplitude of the single channel current seen under patch–clamp and the potential across the channel is linear and is described by Ohm's law. The slope of the current–voltage plot allows measurement of the single-channel conductance, which is reported in units of pico-Siemens (pS). A channel with a conductance of 40 pS would allow a current of 2 pA to flow across a membrane with a potential of 50 mV. To give a sense of how many nAChRs are present on a single muscle cell, we note that a typical pyrantel current (10 μM) in *Brugia malayi* muscle cells is about 100 nA at a membrane potential of −50 mV [14]. This current requires some 50,000 nAChRs to be open simultaneously—the number of nAChRs on nematode muscle is considerable!

Fig. 2.6 shows a histogram of the single-channel conductances of nAChRs observed in a series of experiments on *O. dentatum* muscle cells [15]. The histogram is not a normal distribution, but instead is composed of a number of peaks; this pattern is interpreted as showing that four subtypes of nAChRs are present on these muscle cells, termed the G25 pS, G35 pS, G40 pS and G45 pS subtypes. The single-channel conductance is governed by the molecular structure of the ion channels, so the conductance histogram in Fig. 2.7 suggests that four different subtypes of nAChR exist on muscle cells of *O. dentatum* and produce channels with distinct conductance properties.

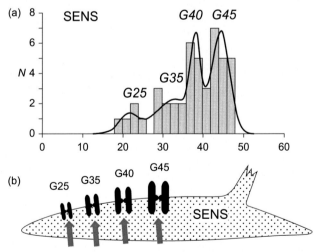

Figure 2.6 (a) Histogram of single channel conductances observed in patches of *O. dentatum* membrane. (b) Note that the histogram is not a normal distribution but has four peaks (G25, G35, G40, and G45) showing the presence of four different nAChR subtypes.

The demonstration of the presence of different nAChR subtypes on muscle cells led to investigations of the effects of anthelmintic nAChR agonists in levamisole-resistant and pyrantel-resistant isolates of *O. dentatum* [15,16]. Fig. 2.7 illustrates the downward spikes of single channel openings in the presence of 30 μM levamisole from the anthelmintic-sensitive isolate,

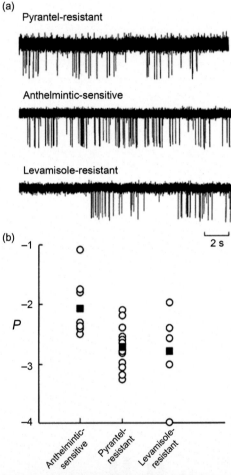

Figure 2.7 (a) Low time resolution (slow) recording of channel opening in representative membrane patches from a pyrantel-resistant *O. dentatum* isolate (top), from an anthelmintic sensitive isolate (middle trace) and from a levamisole-resistant isolate (lower trace). The levamisole concentration used to activate the patches was 30 μM and the membrane potential was −50 mV; channel openings are seen as downward needle-like spikes. (b) Shows the different membrane patch open-channel probabilities (proportion of time the channel is open) at 30 μM levamisole, recorded at −50 mV. Note that the means for pyrantel-resistant and levamisole-resistant isolates are lower than for the anthelmintic-sensitive isolate.

the pyrantel-resistant, and then the levamisole-resistant isolate. The proportion of time the channel was open (P_o) was calculated from experiments on a number of preparations and was displayed as $\log_{10}$ ($P_o + 0.0001$). Log P values closest to 0 reflect the highest P_o values. The pyrantel-resistant isolate had a mean P_o value that was similar to the levamisole-resistant isolate, but both are substantially lower than the value for the sensitive isolate. Thus, in the anthelmintic resistant isolates, the channels open for a shorter period of time than do the channels from the sensitive isolate, meaning that depolarization and Ca^{2+} entry would be reduced along with contraction in the resistant isolate, as would the effect of pyrantel. Interestingly, the effects of pyrantel and levamisole on the distribution of conductances (Fig. 2.7) were different, with levamisole having a major effect on the G35 pS peak and pyrantel having a bigger effect on the G45 pS peak. These results suggest that different subtypes of channel with different subunit composition are differentially sensitive to the two cholinergic anthelmintics.

2.3.4 Contraction Assays Using *A. suum* Muscle Strips

The large parasitic nematode of swine small intestine, *A. suum*, is well-suited for the preparation of muscle strips for experiments on anthelmintic-induced contraction (Fig. 2.8). Application of pyrantel and

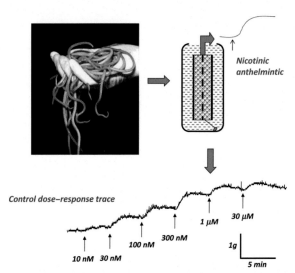

Figure 2.8 Photograph of *Ascaris*-in-hand showing the size and number of worms typically recovered from a host (pig). A muscle flap is prepared from the front region of the parasite and mounted on an isotonic transducer in a bath that allows contractions to be measured in response to the application of nicotinic anthelmintics like pyrantel, levamisole, and bephenium.

other cholinergic anthelmintics produces a graded contraction in *A. suum* muscle strips (Fig. 2.8) that increases in magnitude with agonist concentration [17], including pyrantel, levamisole, and bephenium (Fig. 2.9). Interestingly, paraherquamide, derquantel (Startect), and methyllycaconitine antagonize the effects of these cholinergic agonist anthelmintics in a competitive manner [17] (Figs. 2.9 and 2.10), allowing the potency of the antagonists to be defined by the pK_B value (the negative log of the antagonist dissociation constant: a dissociation constant of 10^{-7} M gives a pK_B of 7.0). The pK_B values (Fig. 2.11) show that effects of nicotine are not well antagonized by paraherquamide ($pK_B = 5.86$), compared to the effects of this drug on responses elicited by levamisole, pyrantel, and bephenium, which are more potently antagonized ($pK_BS = 6.75 - 6.50$). These findings suggest that nicotine activates different receptors than the cholinergic anthelmintics, reinforcing the conclusion that different nAChR subtypes are present on the muscle of *A. suum* and that they are structurally and pharmacologically distinguishable.

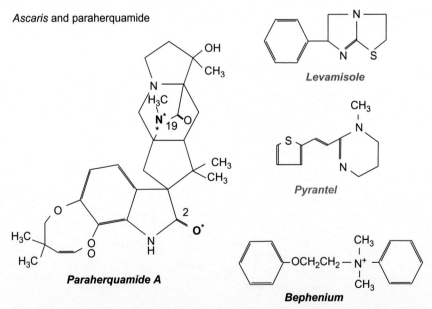

Figure 2.9 Comparison of the chemical structures of the selective nematode nicotinic antagonist paraherquamide A and the agonists levamisole, pyrantel, and bephenium.

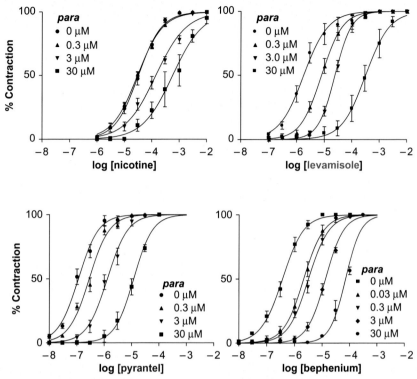

Figure 2.10 % Contraction—concentration response plots for the *Ascaris* muscle strip experiments with paraherquamide A as the antagonist at different concentrations shown against different agonists, nicotine, levamisole, pyrantel, and bephenium. Note that bephenium is antagonized to a greater extent than nicotine by paraherquamide, showing that nicotine and bephenium do not activate the same nAChR subtypes.

2.3.5 Expression of nAChRs in *Xenopus* Oocytes

As noted above, muscle nAChRs activated by the levamisole are thought to consist of five subunits, UNC-63:UNC-38:UNC-29(2):ACR-8 [7,8], which form the receptor ion channel. It has been possible to clone cDNAs encoding the receptor subunits and to express subunits derived from *Haemonchus contortus* [7] and from *O. dentatum* [8] in *Xenopus* oocytes. Functional expression of these receptors is dependent on coexpression of three accessory proteins, UNC-74, UNC-50, and RIC-3. Expression studies of the *H. contortus* subunits found two nAChR subtypes: Hco-L-AChR1, which was most sensitive to levamisole and was composed of the subunits UNC-63:UNC-38:2 (UNC-29):ACR-8; and a

Paraherquamide	nicotine	levamisole	pyrantel	bephenium
pK$_B$ ± s.e.	5.86 ± 0.14[*]	6.61 ± 0.19	6.50 ± 0.11	6.75 ± 0.15

2-deoxyparaherquamide	levamisole	pyrantel	bephenium
pK$_B$ ± s.e.	5.31 ± 0.13	5.64 ± 0.10	6.07 ± 0.13[*]

Figure 2.11 Table of pK$_B$ values (negative log$_{10}$ of the paraherquamide dissociation constant: higher the number means more potent). Paraherquamide is significantly less potent against nicotine than against levamisole, pyrantel, and bephenium, and 2-deoxyparaherquamide (derquantel) is significantly more potent against bephenium than against levamisole and pyrantel. These experiments were interpreted, along with the experiments on the effects of the antagonist methyllycaconitine, to show that there is an N-subtype of nAChR sensitive to ACh, an L-subtype sensitive to levamisole, and a B-subtype sensitive to bephenium.

second, Hco-L-AChR2, which was most sensitive to pyrantel and was composed of an unknown stoichiometric combination of the subunits UNC-63:UNC-38:UNC-29 [7]. The R1 receptor subtype was more sensitive to levamisole and the R2 receptor was more sensitive to pyrantel.

Expression experiments with *O. dentatum* nAChRs [8] followed on from the single channel studies of Robertson et al. [15,16] which revealed that four biophysically different subtypes of nAChR are present on body muscle of the parasite. Additionally, loss of one of these subtypes (G35 pS) was found to be associated with levamisole resistance. Four *O. dentatum* nAChR subunit genes, *Ode-unc-38*, *Ode-unc-63*, *Ode-unc-29* and *Ode-acr-8*, were identified and explored to determine the origin of receptor subtype diversity. When different combinations of subunits were expressed in *Xenopus* oocytes, four pharmacologically distinct types of nAChRs, with different sensitivities to cholinergic anthelmintics, were identified. The pharmacology of these nAChRs varied with the stoichiometric arrangement of the subunits. The minimal requirement for activity was combinations of the subunits Ode-UNC-29, Ode-UNC-63, which made a receptor that was most sensitive to pyrantel, Fig. 2.12. When different combinations of the subunits were tried, three other combinations of subunits produced receptors (Fig. 2.13). The combination of

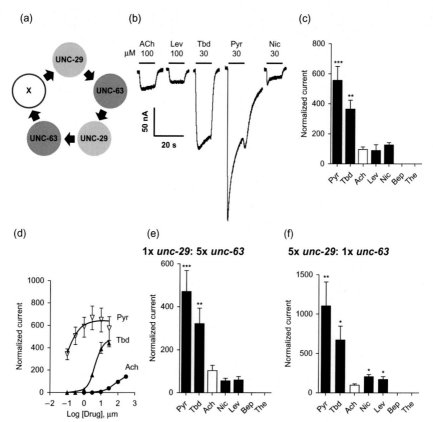

Figure 2.12 Voltage-clamp of *Xenopus* oocytes injected with *O. dentatum* Ode-unc-29 and Ode-unc-63 nAChR subunits. (a) Diagram of possible subunit arrangements of Ode-unc-29 and Ode-unc-63. X represents either UNC-63 or UNC-29. Pyr, pyrantel; Tbd, tribendimidine; ACh, acetylcholine; Nic, nicotine; Bep, bephenium; The, thenium. (b) Representative traces showing inward currents in oocytes injected with 1:1 Ode-unc-29 and Ode-unc-63. (c) Bar chart (mean ± s.e.m.) of agonist-elicited currents in the Ode-(29-63) Pyr-nAChR, (paired *t*-test, **$p < 0.01$, ***$p < 0.001$). All agonist responses normalized to the average 100 μM ACh currents. (d) Dose−response relationships for Pyr (inverted △, $n = 6$), Tbd (▲, $n = 5$) and ACh (•, $n = 6$) in the Ode-(29-63) Pyr-nAChR, ($n =$ number of oocytes). (e) Bar chart (mean ± se) of normalized currents elicited by different agonists in 1:5 Ode-unc-29:Ode-unc-63 injected oocytes. Currents have been normalized to and compared with 100 μM ACh currents (paired *t*-test, **$p < 0.01$, ***$p < 0.001$). (f) Bar chart (mean ± se) of normalized currents elicited by different agonists in oocytes injected with 5:1 Ode-unc-29:Ode-unc-63. Currents normalized to and compared with 100 μM ACh currents (paired *t*-test, *$p < 0.05$, **$p < 0.01$).

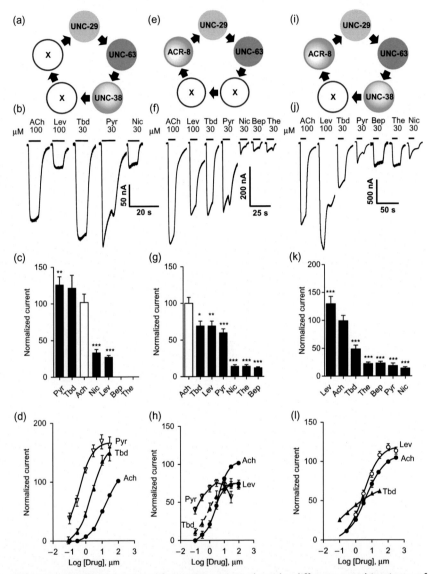

Figure 2.13 Voltage-clamp of oocytes injected with different combinations of the four *O. dentatum* nAChR subunits. (a) Depiction of a possible arrangement of *O. dentatum* UNC-29, UNC-63, and UNC-38. "X" represents any of the subunits. Pyr, pyrantel; Tbd, tribendimidine; ACh, acetylcholine; Nic, nicotine; Bep, bephenium; The, thenium. (b) Representative traces of inward currents elicited by the various agonists in oocytes injected with 1:1:1 Ode-unc-29:Ode-unc-63:Ode-unc-38. Pyr and Tbd were the most potent agonists on this receptor subtype. (c) Bar chart (mean ± se) of currents elicited by the different agonists in the Ode-(29-38-63) Pyr/Tbd-nAChR (paired *(Continued)*

Ode-UNC-29, Ode-UNC-63, Ode-UNC-38, and Ode-ACR-8 subunits behaved like a levamisole receptor and had the same single-channel conductance, 35 pS and 2.4 ms mean open-time properties, as the levamisole-nAChR (G35) subtype previously identified in vivo. Expression of the receptor composed of Ode-UNC-29, Ode-UNC-63, and Ode-UNC-38 was not sensitive to levamisole but was highly sensitive to pyrantel, supporting the hypothesis that distinct nAChR subtypes exist in the parasite, some more sensitive to levamisole, some more sensitive to pyrantel. These studies also showed that the expressed pyrantel receptor (R2 receptor: Ode-UNC-29, Ode-UNC-63, Ode-UNC-38) was more sensitive to the inhibitory effects of derquantel than was the levamisole receptor (R1 receptor: Ode-UNC-29, Ode-UNC-63, Ode-UNC-38, and Ode-ACR-8; Fig. 2.14).

2.3.6 Ca^{2+} Permeability of nAChRs

An effect of increasing external Ca^{2+} from 1 mM to 10 mM [8] on ACh-induced currents in *O. dentatum* nAChRs expressed in oocytes was a positive shift to the right of the current−voltage plot, indicating that the channels are permeable to Ca^{2+}. A shift in reversal potential of 1.7 mV was recorded for the Ode-UNC-29:Ode-UNC-63:Ode-ACR-8 receptors. Using the Goldman Hodgkin Katz constant field equation, the change in reversal potential was used to calculate the Ca^{2+} permeability ratio, P_{Ca}/P_{Na}, of 0.5.

◀ *t*-test, **$p < 0.01$, ***$p < 0.001$). (d) Dose−response of normalized currents versus log concentration for Pyr (inverted △, $n = 6$), Tbd (▲, $n = 6$) and ACh (•, $n = 5$) in the Pyr/Tbd-nAChR. (e) Diagrammatic representation of the three subunits, unc-29, unc-63, and acr-8, injected into oocytes. "X" could be any of the three subunits. (f) Representative traces of inward currents produced by the different agonists in oocytes injected with 1:1:1 Ode-unc-29:Ode-unc-63:Ode-acr-8. (g) Bar chart (mean ± se) of normalized currents elicited by the different agonists in the Ode(29-63-8) receptor subtype. All currents normalized to 100 μM ACh currents; comparisons made with the ACh currents (paired *t*-test, *$p < 0.05$, **$p < 0.01$, ***$p < 0.001$). (h) Dose−response plot of normalized currents versus log. Concentration of Pyr (inverted △, $n = 6$), Tbd (▲, $n = 6$), ACh (•, $n = 6$), and Lev (■, $n = 6$). (i) Representation of a possible arrangement of the four *O. dentatum* subunits injected into *Xenopus* oocytes. (j) Representative traces of inward currents elicited by the different agonists on the Ode(29-63-38-8) or Lev-nAChR. (k) Bar chart (mean ± se) of normalized currents elicited by the different agonists on the Lev-nAChR subtype. Comparisons were made with 100 μM ACh currents, which was used for the normalization (paired *t*-test, ***$p < 0.001$). (l) Dose−response plot of normalized currents against log of Tbd (▲, $n = 6$), ACh (•, $n = 18$) and Lev (○, $n = 5$) concentrations.

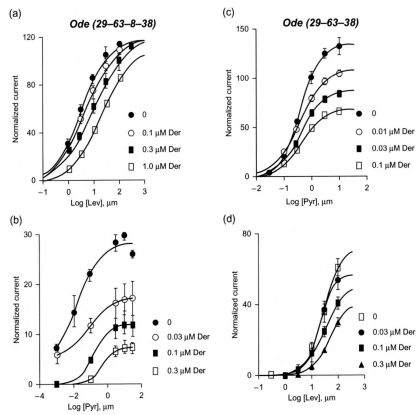

Figure 2.14 Effects of derquantel on levamisole-activated and pyrantel-activated expressed Ode (29-63-8-38), the Lev-nAChR, and on pyrantel-activated and levamisole-activated Ode (29-63-38), the PyR/Tbd-nAChR subtypes. Der, derquantel; Lev, levamisole; Pyr, pyrantel. (a) Antagonistic effects of varying derquantel concentrations on levamisole currents of Ode (29-63-8-38). Levamisole evokes supramaximal normalized currents and derquantel competitively inhibited levamisole currents. (b) Derquantel antagonism of pyrantel currents of Ode (29-63-8-38). Here, derquantel produced mixed noncompetitively competitive antagonism. Pyrantel did not activate supramaximal currents. (c) Antagonism of pyrantel by derquantel on the Ode(29-63-38), Pyr/Tbd-nAChR. Derquantel is a potent noncompetitive antagonist. (d) Derquantel noncompetitively antagonized levamisole responses on the Ode(29-63-38) receptor.

The reversal potential shift for the Ode-UNC-29:Ode-UNC-63:Ode-UNC-38 receptor was similar (1.3 mV), giving a permeability ratio P_{Ca}/P_{Na} of 0.4. For Ode-UNC-29:Ode-UNC-63:Ode-UNC-38:Ode-ACR-8, the shift was 16.0 mV, corresponding to a Ca^{2+} permeability ratio of 10.3. The Ode-UNC-29:Ode-UNC-63:Ode-UNC-38:Ode-ACR-8 receptor is therefore much more permeable to extracellular Ca^{2+} than the other two receptor types, a physiologically significant difference. Ca^{2+} permeability is important because it allows entry of Ca^{2+} and subsequent contraction of the muscle as a result of exposure to pyrantel. The entry of Ca^{2+} through nAChRs produces spastic paralysis and inhibits movement, leading to expulsion of parasites from the GI tract.

2.3.7 Ryanodine Receptors Are Also Involved in the Response to Pyrantel

As documented above, Ca^{2+} enters nematode muscle cells through nAChR channels. The entry of Ca^{2+} through nAChRs can directly activate contraction, but the entry of Ca^{2+} per se also leads to release of Ca^{2+} from intracellular stores in a process mediated by ryanodine receptors, amplifying the effect of channel opening.

These studies used *A. suum* adult anterior body muscle flaps [18,19] that were contracted by application of a cholinergic anthelmintic to examine the role of ryanodine receptors (RyRs) in the excitation−contraction coupling pathway. The maximum force of contraction, g_{max} ($\sim$2 g), was found to be dependent on the extracellular Ca^{2+} concentration, but the anthelmintic EC_{50} was not affected and was insensitive to Ca^{2+}. The maximum force of contraction versus extracellular concentration curve was saturating and well-described by the Michaelis−Menten equation with a K_m value of 1.8 mM. The addition of ryanodine inhibited the maximum force of contraction without affecting the EC_{50}; it only inhibited 44% of the maximum contraction with a $K_i = 40$ nM, revealing a ryanodine-insensitive component of the excitation−contraction pathway. Dantrolene mimicked the effect of ryanodine but was less potent. High concentrations of caffeine (30 mM) produced weak ($\sim$0.2 g) contractions of the body flap preparation, behaving like ryanodine and inhibiting the maximum force of contraction with little effect on anthelmintic EC_{50}s. We conclude that: (1) the force of anthelmintic-induced contractions is dependent on the extracellular Ca^{2+} concentration; and (2) that RyRs play a modulatory role in the anthelmintic-excitation−contraction pathway by affecting the maximum force of contraction without effect on EC_{50}s. Anthelmintic excitation−contraction coupling has at least two pathways: one sensitive to ryanodine and one not; these two pathways can be independently modulated and may be associated with resistance to cholinergic anthelmintics like pyrantel.

2.3.8 Pharmacodynamics

Pyrantel tartrate is well absorbed from the GI tract of pigs and dogs, but not as well in ruminants [3]. The pamoate salt is poorly soluble in water and markedly reduces absorption from the intestine, allowing the drug to reach and sustain effective concentrations in the large intestine, which helps therapeutically in horses and dogs; reduced bioavailability also enhances the therapeutic index. Absorbed pyrantel is quickly metabolized into many compounds [20], which are excreted in the urine (40% of the dose in dogs) with unchanged drug excreted in the feces (principally in ruminants). A useful marker metabolite for monitoring residue levels in ruminants is the hydrolyzed product N-methyl-1,3-propanediamine [21]. Blood concentrations peak at 4–6 h after oral administration, depending on the species and the salt used. Pyrantel citrate is more rapidly absorbed after oral administration to swine, exhibiting higher C_{max} and AUC values with more rapid clearance of pyrantel compared to the pamoate salt [22]. Based on the rapid appearance of pyrantel in the blood, it was suggested [22] that pyrantel is largely absorbed from the upper small intestine. Absorbed pyrantel is excreted with an elimination half-life in plasma of 1–2 h [20], which affords sufficient opportunity for secretion into the distal intestine. This may explain the presence of therapeutic concentrations of pyrantel in the distal intestine.

Morantel, the methyl analog of pyrantel, is reported to be safer and more effective than pyrantel in ruminants after oral administration; significant levels of morantel were not detected in plasma or milk (with one exception) following oral administration of morantel tartrate in goats or cattle [23].

2.4 RESISTANCE TO PYRANTEL AND MORANTEL

2.4.1 Introduction

Anthelmintic resistance in the veterinary arena has been a concern since shortly after the introduction of any new class of drugs, and has consequently been the subject of numerous authoritative reviews. In particular, those by Kelly and Hall [24] and Conder and Campbell [25] illuminate the history of the development of resistance to the tetrahydropyrimidine class of anthelmintics. As of the review by Kelly and Hall in 1979 [24], no reports of field resistance to morantel or pyrantel had appeared [24], but laboratory selection of strains of *H. contortus* resistant to morantel had been achieved [26]. The field situation duplicated this finding in 1979, however, as strains of the sheep parasites *Trichostrongylus colubriformis* and *Ostertagia circumcincta* resistant to morantel tartrate were reported in Australia [26]. The situation had evolved by 1995 [25] after 15 years of use of these drugs in veterinary medicine. In particular, reports of strains of the swine parasite *O. dentatum* and *O. quadrispinulatum* resistant to pyrantel citrate appeared in 1987 [27,28]. A strain of the cattle parasite *Ostertagia ostertagi* resistant to morantel tartrate, selected after use of a rumen bolus, was reported in 1988 [29]. Resistance to pyrantel in small strongyles of horses was thought to be present as early as 1992 [25].

Changes in husbandry practices and competition from alternative anthelmintics, especially the macrocyclic lactone endectocides, have reduced the intensity and extent of use of pyrantel and morantel in many areas of veterinary medicine, and patterns of resistance have evolved as well. These drugs are little used in cattle or small ruminants, and most swine production now involves housed animals with little call for routine anthelmintic treatment. Consequently, concerns now center on pyrantel resistance in horses, companion animals, and humans.

2.4.2 Status of Pyrantel Resistance

Pyrantel resistance in equine cyathostomins was reported in 1996 [30], in large strongyles in 1999 [31], and in *Parascaris equorum* in 2007 [32]. Since then, a number of excellent reviews on pyrantel resistance in equine parasites have appeared [33–38,39]. It can be concluded that pyrantel-resistant large strongyles seem not to have been confirmed as a current problem [40], that pyrantel-resistant cyathostomins have spread globally, and that populations of pyrantel-resistant large strongyles appear so far to be restricted to the United States.

Among companion animals, concerns about pyrantel resistance in populations of the canine hookworm *Ancylostoma caninum* emerged in Australia in 1987 [37]. Further studies in Australia revealed that, by 2007, resistance to pyrantel in populations of this parasite in Brisbane was present and quite profound [41]. Broader surveys of the distribution of this phenotype in Australia have not been reported (see Ref. [42]), nor have pyrantel-resistant canine hookworms been reported from other areas, to the best of our knowledge.

Although pyrantel is approved for human use, as noted above, it is not commonly used intensively for the treatment of human GI nematode infections. However, intensive use in an isolated human settlement in

Australia for control of hookworms (*Ancylostoma duodenale*) apparently led to the selection of resistant strains of this parasite, as a small clinical trial revealed essentially no efficacy (measured by egg reduction) of a standard dose of pyrantel pamoate [43]. This phenotype has not been reported from other sites, and the area in question was treated with albendazole in a campaign that effectively eradicated the parasite locally [44].

It is unsurprising that pyrantel resistance can be readily selected when used intensively. The cases reported in dogs and people represent the best examples of anthelmintic resistance in GI nematodes in these hosts and provide a cautionary tale that should be heeded as mass drug administration campaigns for human GI nematode elimination intensify.

2.4.3 Pharmacology of Resistance

Resistance has been observed in the field relatively soon after the introduction of every class of anthelmintics; this is unsurprising in light of the perceived economic benefits associated with aggressive parasite control, which leads to intensive use of these drugs. Drug resistance can be defined in many ways, but for our purposes, it is a heritable change in susceptibility to a drug such that the concentration— or dose—response curve is shifted to the right in a statistically significant manner. In practical terms, anthelmintic resistance is typically assigned to populations of parasitic nematodes that fail to respond to a therapeutic dose of a drug that is highly efficacious (usually >95%) for that species. Because of the difficulty of working with animals of veterinary importance in laboratory settings and the general inability to maintain target parasite species in laboratory (rodent) hosts, anthelmintic resistant populations are rarely characterized on the basis of percent of a given population that exhibits the phenotype or the quantitative extent of resistance.

As one might expect based simply on the current economics and market share of pyrantel and morantel, relatively little attention has been directed toward understanding the phenotype of pyrantel resistance in parasitic nematodes and its genomic bases. Once we gained an appreciation of the mechanism of action, as detailed above, it was logical to assume that all nAChR agonists would share common mechanisms of receptor-based resistance. Again as illustrated above, the realization that multiple subtypes of nAChRs exist in parasitic nematodes, which vary in sensitivity to agonists, changed our appreciation for the possible complexity of resistance to this class of anthelmintics.

REFERENCES

[1] Austin W, Courtney W, Danilewi JC, Morgan D, Conover L, Howes H, et al. Pyrantel tartrate, a new anthelmintic effective against infections of domestic animals. Nature 1966;212(5067):1273−4.

[2] Jones R.M., Cornwell R.L. Activity of oxantel against *Trichuris suis*. Third international congress of parasitology. Munich; 1974 August 25−31.

[3] Lanusse CL, Alvarez LI, Sallovitz JM, Mottier ML, Sanchez Bruni SF. Antinematodal agents. In: Riviere JE, Papich MG, editors. Veterinary pharmacology and therapeutics. 9th ed. Ames, IA: Wiley-Blackwell; 2009. p. 1079−83.

[4] Keiser J, Utzinger J. Efficacy of current drugs against soil-transmitted helminth infections: systemic review and meta-analysis. J Am Med Assoc 2008;299(16): 1937−48.

[5] Dashper S, O'Brien-Simpson N, Liu S, Paolini R, Mitchell H, Walsh K, et al. Oxantel disrupts polymicrobial biofilm development of periodontal pathogens. Antimicrob Agents Chemother 2014;58(1):378−85.

[6] Aubry ML, Cowell P, Davey MJ, Shevde S. Aspects of the pharmacology of a new anthelmintic: pyrantel. Br J Pharmacol 1970;38:332−44.

[7] Boulin T, Fauvin A, Charvet C, Cortet J, Cabaret J, Bessereau J-L, et al. Functional Reconstitution of *Haemonchus contortus* acetylcholine receptors in *Xenopus* oocytes provides mechanistic insights into levamisole resistance. Brit J Pharm 2011;164 (5):1421−32.

[8] Buxton SK, Charvet CL, Neveu C, Cabaret J, Cortet J, Peineau N, et al. Investigation of acetylcholine receptor diversity in a nematode parasite leads to characterization of tribendimidine- and derquantel-sensitive nAChRs. PLoS Pathog 2014;10(1):e1003870.

[9] Robertson SJ, Pennington AJ, Evans AM, Martin RJ. The action of pyrantel as an agonist and an open-channel blocker at acetylcholine receptors in isolated *Ascaris suum* muscle vesicles. Eur J Pharmacol 1994;271(2-3):273−82.

[10] Rayes D, De Rosa MJ, Spitzmaul G, Bouzat C. The anthelmintic pyrantel acts as a low efficacious agonist and an open-channel blocker of mammalian acetylcholine receptors. Neuropharmacology 2001;41(2):238−45.

[11] Bartos M, Rayes D, Bouzat C. Molecular determinants of pyrantel selectivity in nicotinic receptors. Mol Pharmacol 2006;70(4):1307−18.

[12] Wu TY, Smith CM, Sine SM, Levandoski MM. Morantel allosterically enhances channel gating of neuronal nicotinic acetylcholine alpha 3 beta 2 receptors. Mol Pharmacol 2008;74(2):466−75.

[13] Cesa LC, Higgins CA, Sando SR, Kuo DW, Levandoski MM. Specificity determinants of allosteric modulation in the neuronal nicotinic acetylcholine receptor: a fine line between inhibition and potentiation. Mol Pharmacol 2012;81(2):239−49.

[14] Robertson AP, Buxton SK, Martin RJ. Whole-cell patch-clamp recording of nicotinic acetylcholine receptors of *Brugia malayi* muscle. Parasitol Int 2013;62(6): 616−18.

[15] Robertson AP, Bjorn HE, Martin RJ. Resistance to levamisole resolved at the single-channel level. FASEB J 1999;13(6):749−60.

[16] Robertson AP, Bjorn HE, Martin RJ. Pyrantel resistance alters nematode nicotinic acetylcholine receptor single-channel properties. Eur J Pharmacol 2000;394(1):1−8.

[17] Robertson AP, Clark CL, Burns TA, Thompson DP, Geary TG, Trailovic SM, et al. Paraherquamide and 2-deoxy-paraherquamide distinguish cholinergic receptor subtypes in *Ascaris* muscle. J Pharmacol Exp Ther 2002;302(3):853−60.

[18] Robertson AP, Clark CL, Martin RJ. Levamisole and ryanodine receptors (I): a contraction study in *Ascaris suum*. Mol Biochem Parasitol 2010;171(1):1−7.

[19] Puttachary S, Robertson AP, Clark CL, Martin RJ. Levamisole and ryanodine receptors. II: an electrophysiological study in *Ascaris suum*. Mol Biochem Parasitol 2010;171(1):8—16.

[20] Faulkner JK, Figdor SK, Monro AM, Schach von Wittenau M, Stopher DA, Wood BA. The comparative metabolism of pyrantel in five species. J Sci Food Agric 1972;23(1):79—91.

[21] Ho C, Lee WO, Wong YT. Determination of N-methyl-1,3-propanediamine in bovine muscle by liquid chromatography with triple quadrupole and ion trap tandem mass spectrometry detection. J Chromatgr A 2012;1235:103—14.

[22] Bjorn H, Hennessy DR, Friis C. The kinetic disposition of pyrantel citrate and pamoate and their efficacy against pyrantel-resistant *Oesophagostomum dentatum* in pigs. Int J Parasitol 1996;26(12):1375—80.

[23] McKellar QA, Scott EW, Baxter P, Anderson LA, Bairden K. Pharmacodynamics, pharmacokinetics and faecal persistence of morantel in cattle and goats. J Vet Pharmacol Ther 1993;16(1):87—92.

[24] Kelly JD, Hall CA. Resistance of animal helminths to anthelmintics. Adv Pharmacol Chemother 1979;16:89—128.

[25] Conder GA, Campbell WC. Chemotherapy of nematode infections of veterinary importance, with special reference to drug resistance. Adv Parasitol 1995;35:1—83.

[26] Le Jambre LF, Southcott WH, Dash KM. Resistance of selected lines of *Haemonchus contortus* to thiabendazole, morantel tartrate and levamisole. Int J Parasitol 1976;6:217—22.

[27] Roepstorff A, Bjørn H, Nansen P. Resistance of *Oesophagostomum* spp. in pigs to pyrantel citrate. Vet Parasitol 1987;24:229—39.

[28] Bjørn H, Roepstorff A, Nansen P, Waller P. Reistance to levamisole and cross-resistance between pyrantel and levamisole in *Oesophagostomum quadrispinulatum* and *Oesophagostomum dentatum* of pigs. Vet Parasitol 1990;37:21—30.

[29] Borgsteede FHM. The difference between two strains of *Ostertagia ostertagi* in resistance to morantel tartrate. Int J Parasitol 1988;18:499—502.

[30] Chapman MR, French DD, Monahan CM, Klei TR. Identification and characterization of a pyrantel pamoate resistant cyathostome population. Vet Parasitol 1996;66:205—12.

[31] Coles GC, Brown SN, Trembath CM. Pyrantel-resistant large strongyles in racehorses. Vet Rec 1999;145(14):408.

[32] Craig TM, Diamond PL, Ferwerda NS, Thompson JA. Evidence of ivermectin resistance by *Parascaris equorum* on a Texas horse farm. J Equine Vet Sci 2007;27:67—71.

[33] von Samson-Himmelstjerna G. Anthelmintic resistance in equine parasites—detection, potential clinical relevance and implications for control. Vet Parasitol 2012;185:1—8.

[34] Reinemeyer CR. Anthelmintic resistance in non-strongylid parasites of horses. Vet Parasitol 2012;185:9—15.

[35] Neilsen MK, Reinemeyer CR, Donecker JM, Leathwick DM, Marchiondo AA, Kaplan RM. Anthelmintic resistance in equine parasites—current evidence and knowledge gaps. Vet Parasitol 2014;204:55—63.

[36] Matthews JB. Anthelmintic resistance in equine nematodes. Int J Parasitol: Drugs Drug Resist 2014;4:310—15.

[37] Jackson R, Lance D, Townsend K. Isolation of anthelmintic resistant *Ancylostoma caninum*. N Z Vet J 1987;35:215—16.

[38] Sangser NC, Whitlock HV, Russ IG, Gunawan M, Griffin DL, Kelly JD. *Trichostrongylus colubriformis* and *Ostertagia circumcincta* resistant to levamisole, morantel tartrate and thiabendazole: occurrence of field strains. Res Vet Sci 1979;27:106—10.

[39] Peregrine AS, Molento MB, Kaplan RM, Nielsen MK. Anthelmintic resistance in important parasites of horses: does it really matter? Vet Parasitol 2014;201:1–8.

[40] Kaplan RM. Anthelmintic resistance in nematodes of horses. Vet Res 2002;33 (5):491–507.

[41] Kopp SR, Coleman GT, McCarthy JS, Kotze AC. Phenotypic characterization of two *Ancylostoma caninum* isolates with different susceptibilities to the anthelmintic pyrantel. Antimicrob Agents Chemother 2008;52:3980–6.

[42] Kopp SR, Coleman GT, Traub RJ, McCarthy JS, Kotze AC. Acetylcholine receptor subunit genes from *Ancylostoma caninum*: altered transcription patterns associated with pyrantel resistance. Int J Parasitol 2009;39:435–41.

[43] Reynoldson JA, Behnke JM, Pallant LJ, Macnish MG, Gilbert F, Giles S, et al. Failure of pyrantel in treatment of human hookworm infections (*Ancylostoma duodenale*) in the Kimberley region of North West Australia. Act Trop 1997;68:301–12.

[44] Thompson RCA, Reynoldson JA, Garrow SC, McCarthy JS, Behnke JM. Towards the eradication of hookworm in an isolated Australian community. Lancet 2001; 357:770–1.

CHAPTER 3

The Safety of Pyrantel, Oxantel, and Morantel

C.D. Mackenzie
Department of Pathobiology and Diagnostic Investigation, Michigan State University, East Lansing, MI, United States

3.1 INTRODUCTION

The purpose of this present discussion is to cover the safety and clinical toxicological aspects of three tetrahydropyrimidines, pyrantel (PY), oxantel (OX), and morantel (MO). These three agents, especially the first, have been in common use in veterinary and human medicine for some time. PY was discovered in 1966 [1] and, in what is testament to the safe nature of at least the first of these three drugs, since that time there have been relatively few reports of serious adverse events. In fact the literature related to PY, which is much more extensive than that of the other two agents, is largely focused on efficacy and function. It is not the purpose of this discussion here to discuss these agents in relation to details of their use and their pharmacology unless it is relevant to the safety of the agent.

In discussing the safety of drugs used in humans and animals it is important to note that by virtue of their mode of action on a specific target system in the parasite there is often, at least the potential, of a corresponding effect on the host due to similarity in the pharmaco–physiologic targets in the two species. Thus any discussion of the safety of a chemotherapeutic agent necessitates a careful consideration of the interaction between the drug and the host being treated. With a number of drugs there are significant variations in their response to the drug and the possibility of adverse reactions due to differences in age, infection status, and the presence of other chemotherapeutic treatments being used at the same time. A central principle in the use of toxic drugs whose primary pharmacological action on the target parasite also occurs in the host's tissues and organs is to determine the relative differences in these effects between the two species, and the outcomes of these actions. Thus a discussion of the safety of a chemotherapeutic agent can be discussed from a number of angles. These include

Pyrantel Parasiticide Therapy in Humans and Domestic Animals.
DOI: http://dx.doi.org/10.1016/B978-0-12-801449-3.00014-4
47

considering the direct effects on the individual being treated by the drug itself, secondly the effects that result from being administered in conjunction with other agents that also act on this target, toxic events that are host-dependent (eg, age-dependence), and lastly toxicity that is cumulative (ie, due to repeated use of the agent in question).

This group of drugs have been used much more extensively in the veterinary world than in human medicine and currently there are also differences in the recommendations for their use in these two medical areas, with human medicine often being more understandably restrictive, due perhaps to the lack of investigatory evidence in human medicine; for example, their use in the very young is more limited in human medicine. There are certainly differences in the pharmacodynamics of these drugs between the species due to anatomical and physiological differences but it is clear that these agents are indeed useful in many species.

This group of drugs, the tetrahydropyrimidines, act on the nervous system of worms by inhibiting the central agent in the neurotransmitter system, acetyl cholinesterase, and causing an interruption and alteration to the impulses moving from nerves to muscles, and between neurones within the CNS; there is an interruption to cholinergic brain synapses. This action of the cholinergic anthelmintics has been well reviewed in detail by Martin et al. [2]. The overall effect of this action is manifested physically by altering the control of movement by the target worms, which can cause them to be expelled as they are unable to maintain their environment, to be paralyzed and subsequently to be rejected or die. The three drugs discussed in this chapter all essentially act this way although their effectiveness at this outcome differs somewhat due to differences in the physico-chemical and pharmacological properties of each primary agent and its salt.

3.2 PYRANTEL

PY [1] is the most used, and the best described, of the three agents in terms of its use, action, and importantly here, its safety. It is in general terms, if used as directed, a safe drug in virtually all species (including humans), and is reported to induce, at worst, relatively mild reactions such as vomiting, headache, and mild intestinal disturbances. It is active on a number of intestinal worms, and is better than many other drugs against the often difficult to treat intestinal parasite, *Trichuris* sp. PY is an antinematodal thiophene, a nicotinic receptor agonist, and is commonly used for the prevention of intestinal parasites in small animal pets, and in humans as a relatively effective agent against whipworms and other intestinal nematodes. However, it should also be noted that it does not work with *Necator americanus* and is therefore not the panacea drug [3].

3.2.1 Mode of Action

Its mode of action, which is similar to that of another of this group under discussion here, MO, and like levamisole, elicits spastic muscle paralysis in the target helminth due to prolonged activation of the excitatory nicotinic acetylcholine receptors on body wall muscle [2]. Nicotinic acetylcholine receptors are widely expressed in nematode nervous systems both at the neuromuscular junctions on the muscle cells and in the neurons themselves [1]. PY pamoate acts as a depolarizing neuromuscular blocking agent, thereby causing sudden contraction, followed by paralysis, of the helminths. This has the result of causing the worm to "lose its grip" on the intestinal wall and be passed out of the system by natural processes. PY is more potent than levamisole in its effect on muscle contractility and membrane potential effecting somatic nicotinic cholinergic transmission; $1-10$ μmol of PY causes spastic contraction and sustained paralysis. PY is faster acting than levamisole in its effects and causes membrane depolarization at the muscle membrane. Important differences have been shown in its effect on *Haemonchus* and the mammalian (rat) host targets, with PY being more active on the worm than on the animal [4]. Since PY is poorly absorbed by the host's intestine, the host is unaffected by the small dosage of medication used.

The forms of PY used commercially can differ in their pharmacodynamic properties and this can affect their safety profile in some cases primarily due to their differential absorption into the blood from the gut. The time taken to be absorbed can on the one hand reduce the time for an effect on the intestinal worms residing in the gut, and on the other hand rapid absorption can expose the host more readily to toxicity to the agent. For example, PY tartrate is more soluble in water than PY pamoate with the consequent higher absorption of the tartrate into the blood resulting in a higher potential for toxicity. There is better absorption from the gut of monogastric animals compared with ruminants. Thus the amount of time the drug remains in the intestine, and able to damage parasites that are present in the gut, is a central factor here, especially for those parasites present further down the gastrointestinal tract such as in the large bowel, such as *Trichuris* sp.

In general, both in animals and humans PY is poorly absorbed by the gut after oral administration and in safety terms is generally well tolerated by these species. Because of the relatively slow development of the intestinal barrier in many species there is higher degree of toxicity in young animals compared with adults. Calves, for example, treated with PY tartrate at doses more than 200 mg/kg showed ataxia (uncoordinated movements), whereas mature cattle tolerate much higher levels. Decisions relating to the optimal form of the drug, that is, the pamoate salt versus the tartrate, or the citrate, are affected by these properties. In nonruminants, for example, the pamoate form is preferred as it is less absorbent and thus allows for higher safety margins. Safety margins (the range between the minimal therapeutic dose and the minimal toxic dose of a drug) of PY pamoate are in most species greater than 10 (~15 in cattle and ~20 in horses).

PY is metabolized relatively quickly by the liver. In ruminants (cattle) some 70% of the administered dose is usually excreted through feces mostly as unchanged drug. In contrast, in monogastric animals (dogs and pigs) around 40% of the drug is excreted through the urine as breakdown metabolites. Although there is evidence that PY is partially excreted in the milk of animals the situation with regard to human breast milk is unclear. Not only is the status of the treated individual's gut wall important regarding the absorption of PY, the actual contents of the gut (ie, the diet), as well as any specific physiological mechanisms pertaining to that species are also important; thus the diet can have an important influence. For example in pigs, PY citrate given with a fiber-poor diet passes more slowly through the stomach, with consequently a longer absorption period, and a resulting increase in anthelmintic bioavailability. In dogs, administration of PY with the food also increases the time in the stomach and its bioavailability. Thus in terms of safety issues the question of both the pathophysiological status of the gut (normal vs underlying pathology), as well as the timing of treatment in relation to food intake must at least be considered; although it should be noted that many commercial instructions for the drug indicate that the drug can be taken safely with or without food. This may be true but is also true that the effectiveness of the drug may be affected by the diet.

An important biochemical investigation showed that there was no effect of PY on P450 reduction nor any active induction of cytochrome P450 [5] suggesting that PY is, in the bigger scheme of things, a very safe drug from the biochemical angle. Interestingly this was not the case with albendazole and P450, where there was an effect seen; this difference may reflect differences in drug metabolism and clearance of drugs in the treated individuals between these two very commonly used drugs in humans. PY has no effect on antioxidant enzymes, and no effect on the activity of antioxidant enzymes induced in animals that were poisoned with dimethoate [6], all of which supported the use of PY as a safe agent for use in mammals.

There is contrary evidence as to the effect of PY on the anatomy of the worms. In one study PY did not induce any detectable physical changes in the ultrastructure of trichostrongyles [7]; this differs from ivermectin, thiabendazole, and levamisole, all of which induce changes. In contrast, a study on *Toxocara* using PY at levels ranging from 23.6 μg to 2360 μg/mL medium showed that the intestinal hypodermis, and muscle cells are physically affected by the drug [8]. Incubation time, that is, exposure, seemed in these studies to be more important than concentration of the drug in inducing an effect. Adult worms are believed to ingest PY orally whereas preadult *Toxocara* take it in through the body surface. This study also suggested that adult worms initially limit ingestion of the drug for the first 4 h before then digesting large amounts of the drug; in contrast the preadult forms appear to absorb the drug continuously for the first 14 h. The changes in morphology brought about by PY, and indeed OX and MO, is probably an area of investigation that could be enhanced by further morphological and in situ molecular studies.

There is conflicting data concerning the effect of PY on genetic targets. Mutagenicity studies using *Salmonella typhimurium* indicated that PY was relatively safe [9], but, in contrast, another study showed that PY pamoate increased sperm head abnormalities in mice [10] and suggested that it might therefore be mutagenic; levamisole, albendazole, mebendazole, and thiabendazole did not do this. Others have suggested that PY may induce gene conversion or aneuploidy [11], and other larval test systems using PY with *Haemonchus* and *Ostertagia circumcincta* [12] could be used to study both morphological and genetic changes. This is a difficult and important area of toxicological investigation today with anthelmintics, particular with new agents and repurposed agents, which is difficult in part because of the aspects of relative risk that are involved in the assessment of any apparently negative findings.

3.2.2 Usage

PY remains a safe and useful anthelmintic drug that has a place in the management of nematode infections in human and veterinary medicine.

PY has a positive benefit—risk profile for use in humans, and it is retained on the current list of the WHO Model List of Essential Medicines as one of the six intestinal anthelmintics, and is listed in the WHO Model Formulary [13]. PY is generally used against strongyles, pinworms, and roundworms, in regimens ranging from a single dose to 3 days of daily doses; it is used as an oral dose of 11 mg of base per kilogram base body weight and double this (22 mg/kg) for the treatment of tapeworms; it is used up to a maximum of 1 g. The dosage used is the same for children as for adults. PY pamoate (under US Pharmacopeia) or PY embonate (under European Pharmacopoeia) is used as a deworming agent for intestinal nematodes including the treatment of most species of hookworms (although there is some contrary evidence regarding its efficacy against *N. americanus*) and roundworms. However, it has been suggested that it may not be effective against all strains of a particular helminth. It also is used to treat tissue nematode infection such as trichinosis in humans.

It is very commonly used in veterinary medicine in small and large animals. PY pamoate is indicated for the removal and control of mature infections of large strongyles (*Strongylus vulgaris, S. edentatus, S. equinus*), small strongyles, pinworms (*Oxyuris equi*), large roundworms (*Parascaris equorum*), and tapeworms (*Anoplocephala perfoliata*) in horses and ponies [14,15]. Studies with PY in goats showed it to be effective against *Haemonchus contortus* (96% effective) and similarly with *Teladorsagia circumcincta* but not against *Trichostrongylus colubriformis* where it was only around 60% effective [16]; it is also effective against similar worms in sheep [17].

3.2.3 Safety and Toxicity

The side effects seen with PY are most often related to the intestine (eg, vomiting and nausea) or to more general symptoms (such as headache), and these can occur at therapeutic doses. Thus it is strongly recommended that PY is not administered to sick or otherwise weak and infirm individuals. Importantly it should be noted that a damaged gastrointestinal mucosa might enhance absorption and increase subsequent toxicity. In studies addressing the pharmacodynamics of PY in humans—where the peak plasma concentrations reached 36 ng/mL at 2 h after 750 mg of PY—abdominal discomfort was noted in one of nine people and dizziness also in one of nine [18]. Other studies have shown a complete lack of side reactions despite high efficacy [19].

There is extensive and established safety experience with PY in several countries. The drug has been well-studied and adverse reaction profiles well documented. Even though there are several adverse reactions reported in association with its use in the WHO database, the drug is still widely used for hookworm infections, enterobiasis, and tissue nematode infections. Importantly the most frequent adverse reactions to PY relate to the gastrointestinal system and are mild. There is no information to suggest an unfavorable safety profile of the drug under current conditions of use and the drug remains a safe and useful anthelmintic drug that has a place in the management of nematode infections. The adverse reactions to PY recorded in the Uppsala Monitoring Centre (UMC)/WHO database for humans list gastrointestinal system disorders as predominating with mild systemic changes also being fairly common, although these are three times more commonly reported than those related to the nervous system and the skin and appendages. The French Pharmacovigilance database records 10 adverse drug reports during PY treatment for ascariasis [4], pinworm [5], and one for an unspecified helminth infection. These reports included four cases of nausea, vomiting and flatulence; pruritus and urticaria (two cases); and a case each of dizziness, headache, and hypotonia, and one case of paraesthesia associated with ataxia and weakness. Two hundred and three adverse drug reaction case reports involving 468 adverse reactions associated with PY use are present in the WHO ADR database. The majority of these reports originate from Australia where there is an active pharmacovigilance system. The main organs and systems affected are the gastrointestinal tract, the body as a whole, the central and peripheral nervous systems, as well as skin and appendages.

As stated above, PY may cause side effects, albeit usually mild, that include vomiting, diarrhea, loss of appetite, stomach cramps, stomach pain, straining and pain during bowel movements. The more systemic side effects associated with PY are also generally mild and include headache, dizziness, drowsiness, insomnia, rash, and elevated liver enzymes. Drug allergies are also listed, although documented evidence for this presentation is hard to find. Whether the inability to tolerate the drug in those that do react is a true allergy or not is unclear. There may be true allergic reactions to one or more of the other components present in a PY medication, especially in sensitive species like cats. In all likelihood allergies are listed as a precautionary statement rather than defined common occurrence, and could occur, as with any drug treatment, in rare cases. Dogs who exhibit sensitivities to other medications may also have a problem with PY pamoate for general intestinal sensitivity issues that are not true allergies. However, if true allergic reactions to the medication occur they would present as the common signs and symptoms of allergies such as hives, itching, and swelling.

Spastic (tetanic) paralyzing agents, in particular PY pamoate, may induce complete intestinal obstruction in a heavy worm load [4]. This obstruction when it occurs is usually in the form of a worm impaction and happens when a very small, but heavily parasitized, animal is treated and tries to pass a large number of dislodged worms at once. Worms usually pass in normal stool or with diarrhea, straining, and occasional vomiting.

One of the earliest studies on the effects of PY on the host was carried out in greyhound dogs and showed the blood levels of enzymes were normal after treatment except for serum alkaline phosphatase (SAP) levels, which decreased; other standard serum enzymes such as serum glutamic-oxaloacetic transaminase, serum glutamic-pyruvic transaminase, and serum cholinesterase remained within normal levels [20]. This reduction SAP was similar to that seen with piperazine use in puppies. This differential effect on puppies compared to adult dogs involving this enzyme has not been fully explained but may be related to the presence of actively growing bones in these animals. PY causes a decrease in the accumulation of vitamin C in the liver at one-fifth of the LD_{50} in rats [21] (Table 3.1).

There is an unusual case of massive proteinuria in a 4-year-old boy with a history of oxyuriasis and treatment with parental permeate 7 days before the development of urino-pathology [22]. This paper was written to alert pediatricians and suggested there might have been a nephrotic syndrome complex in this single case; however, this is an isolated case and cannot be taken as a typical response to the use of PY even if it was in fact initiated here by the use of the drug.

Table 3.1 The LD_{50} levels for the three tetrahydropyrimidines, pyrantel, oxantel, and morantel in different species

Species	Agent	LD_{50} acute (mg/kg)
Rats and mice	Pyrantel tartrate (po)	170
Rats	Pyrantel pamaote	>5000
Dog	Pyrantel pamaote	>690
Rats	Oxantel pamoate	980
Mice	Oxantel pamoate	300
Rabbit	Oxantel pamoate	3200
Mice	Morantel tartrate	5000
Rats	Morantel tartrate	926

In summary, it is clear that there is an extensive and well-documented safety record with PY in several countries and all the adverse reactions seen are well documented. Even though there are in fact several types of adverse reactions recorded in association with its use in the WHO database, the drug is still widely recommended for hookworm infections, enterobiasis, and tissue nematode infections. As discussed above the most frequent adverse reactions to PY relate to the gastrointestinal system and are mild. There is no information to suggest an unfavorable safety profile of the drug under current conditions where it is used that would limit its further use, and the drug remains a safe and useful anthelmintic drug that has a place in the management of nematode infections.

3.2.4 Species Differences

There is considerable variability in susceptibility to developing toxic events between the species, and this depends on the form of PY used. Horses for example tolerate PY pamoate better than the PY tartrate; these animals tolerated 75 mg/kg PY tartrate well, but at 100 mg/kg deaths can occur. In dogs studied for subchronic toxicity, animals treated at 20 mg/kg/day during 3 months did not show toxic symptoms, but at 50 mg/kg/day they showed symptoms of intoxication. Kittens 4- to 6-week-old treated at 300 mg/kg/day during 3 days did not show any clinical symptoms. There was no toxicity in chickens with PY tartrate [23]. PY paste has been used in treatment for tapeworm in horses with no adverse effects [24]; the NOAEL level in this study was 132 mg/kg after 6 days (UID 6 days), indicating that 13.2 mg/kg is safe in this species.

PY is generally thought to be safe for the environment if used as directed and is not detrimental to coprophagous insects. It is not used to date in crop pesticides.

3.2.5 Use in Combination with Other Drugs

As early as 1972 it was realized that there is a danger from combining drugs that affected nicotinic receptors in conjunction with cholinergic drugs and with organophosphate compounds (which are anticholinergic agents) [25]. However, PY is often used safely in combination with benzimidazoles (including its prodrugs) and/or praziquantel, ivermectin, and OX, particularly in dogs and cats. Incompatibilities or antagonistic effects have not been reported with use in these species although increases in mild side effects could be expected. Importantly there are combinations that are contraindicated: PY and piperazine have an antagonistic effect on certain parasites and should not be administered simultaneously, since one compound can neutralize the effect of the other, at least in species where this has been studied (*Ascaris* sp.). PY must not be administered together with levamisole or MO, because they all share the same mechanism of action and therefore the same toxic effects. Organophosphates and diethylcarbamazine are also inhibitors of acetyl cholinesterase and can enhance the toxicity of PY.

The safety and efficacy of a combination of PY plus OX plus praziquantel has been assessed in dogs with animals treated with either two times the recommended therapeutic dose, with six times the recommended therapeutic dose, or twice with the recommended dose on three consecutive days [26]; no difference in the blood parameters and no abnormal clinical findings were detected. The only adverse clinical effect seen was in two of the dogs treated with six times the recommended treatment dose who did have bouts of vomiting but these lasted less than 2 days.

PY may react with organophosphates, diethylcarbamazine citrate, levamisole, MO, and piperazine. Levamisole, a nicotine-like compound that may interact with PY, can cause nicotinic toxicosis with a wide range of physiological and pathophysiological responses including hepatic necrosis and splenic congestion [27]. Giving 25 mg/kg of PY an hour before levamisole increased the toxicity of the levamisole [28].

3.2.6 Contraindications

PY is considered safe to use in nursing animals [5] but is not recommended for use during pregnancy in humans. The concern with the use of PY in neonates in all likelihood is based on differences in the intestine in terms of absorption compared to older individuals. The recommendation given is that it not be used in humans younger than 2 years of age; however, in a somewhat contrasting situation it is one of the most most common antiworming agents currently used in puppies and kittens. PY pamoate is considered a pregnancy category C drug for use during pregnancy for humans, but is in category A for canines and felines. The PY pamoate definition as a pregnancy category C is where the FDA has that noted that in animal reproduction studies there have been adverse effects on the fetus and that there are no adequate and well-controlled studies in humans. Data on the use of PY pamoate in pregnant women are limited, however, the potential benefits may warrant use of the drug in pregnant women despite potential risks. In mass treatment programs for which WHO has determined that the benefit of treatment outweighs the risk, WHO allows use of PY pamoate in the second and third trimesters of pregnancy, acknowledging that the effects of PY on birth outcome are not certain. The risk of treatment in pregnant women who are known to have an infection needs to be balanced with the risk of disease progression in the absence of treatment.

It is not known whether PY pamoate is excreted in breast milk. WHO now classifies PY pamoate as compatible with breastfeeding, although data on the use of PY pamoate during lactation are limited and documents often still carry warnings against treating women who are breast-feeding with PY. As it is poorly absorbed from the gastrointestinal tract and very low levels are detected in breast milk it is likely to be safe. There are no pediatric specific problems documented in the literature and the drug is not as yet fully recommended for use in children less than 1 year of age; although, as mentioned above PY, is safe for use in pregnant and nursing domestic animals. Puppies automatically receive PY pamoate as a prophylactic. Current WHO guidance on preventive chemotherapy, does indicate that PY might be used in children aged 1 year and older during mass treatment programs without diagnosis. However, as a matter of principle, PY should not be used in conjunction with other dewormers unless advised as being a safe practice by published accepted clinical studies or by reputable companies' official recommendations.

It has been reported that piperazine may counteract the anthelmintic effect of PY [5]. Theophylline may have dangerous side effects when taken during therapy with PY; a report exists in the literature of an interaction between PY and theophylline that led to an increase in serum theophylline levels [29]; other drugs used to treat infections caused by worms may also decrease the effectiveness of PY.

Other areas related to safety that have not yet been fully investigated include drug resistance and effects on nutrition of those treated. Resistance to PY has been described to develop with treatment of cyathostomes in ponies where there was a reduction of 62−80% of efficacy with 6.6 mg/kg dosing [30]; there also appeared to be dual resistance to the benzimidazole oxybendazole in this case. The need to consider the possibility of this form of problem developing has been emphasized by other authors [31]. PY causes a decrease in the accumulation of vitamin C in the liver at one-fifth of the LD_{50} in rats [21].

3.2.7 Antidote and Treatment of PY

The antidote for PY toxicity is atropine, should one be needed. Atropine is a competitive antagonist of the muscarinic acetylcholine receptors. However, it should be noted that atropine is itself incapacitating at doses of more than 10 mg/human individual. For symptomatic bradycardia, the usual dosage is 0.5−1 mg IV push, which may be repeated every 3−5 min up to a total dose of 3 mg (maximum 0.04 mg/kg).

PY remains a safe and useful anthelmintic drug that has a place in the management of nematode infections in virtually all species.

3.3 OXANTEL

OX the second of this group of tetrahydropyrimidines has been less used and less documented than PY, but nevertheless it remains a most useful anthelmintic drug and has some minor differences from the other two in this group discussed in this chapter.

3.3.1 Action

There is a difference in OX's action compared with PY and MO and this is thought to be due to the action on a different subtype of cholinergic receptors, the N-subtype receptors, which are sensitive to nicotine and methyridine; PY and MO act on the L-subtype which is sensitive to levamisole [32].

3.3.2 Usage

Dogs can be safely treated with combination drugs that include OX with PY and praziquantel, with this combination being highly efficacious against a range of parasites of dogs; achieving more than 97% efficacy with *Toxocara canis*, *Ancylostoma caninum*, *Toxascaris leonina*, *Trichuris vulpis*, *Uncinaria stephocephala*, *Taenia* spp., and *Dipylidium caninum* [33]. OX has been proposed as a useful agent in aiding the usually difficult task of controlling *Trichuris* sp. infections in humans and animals. In a study carried out on Pemba Island in Africa comparing combinations of various anthelmintic agents on *Trichuris trichuria* and other intestinal helminths in children, using 40 mg/kg of albendazole given with 20 mg/kg OX pamoate, showed that the number of children cured and the reduction in egg counts where OX was included was superior to other drug combinations [34].

3.3.3 Safety and Toxicity

The most common intoxication symptoms caused by OX poisoning are similar to the adverse reactions during therapy with PY, namely nausea, vomiting, diarrhea, and loss of appetite. Dogs tolerate OX very well, due to its low toxicity and its slow absorption into blood after oral administration; the pamoate salt form of OX has a safety margin in dogs of approximately 15. Humans can suffer from mild reactions following treatment with OX. In the study on Pemba [34], 20% of children showed some form of side effect although they were only mild. Abdominal cramps were seen in 18.2% of the children taking OX plus albendazole, which was higher than in any of the other combination groups that did not include OX. Headache was seen in 10.9% of the children taking OX plus albendazole which was again a higher level than that seen in any of the other groups; however as noted above the group with OX was more parasitologically effective. In a second study on Pemba it was noted that OX had a low efficacy against hookworm and *Ascaris*, and recorded again the fact that mild adverse events occur in children who received OX, in this example 30.9% of those treated [35].

3.3.4 Species Differences

There is little information available on the effects of OX on the environment, as its fate and general toxicity in this area of biology have not been investigated. It is currently not being used in crop pesticides, and it is generally felt that its correct use on dogs and cats is unlikely to be detrimental for the environmental, including not having any significant effect on coprophagous insects.

3.3.5 Antidote for Intoxication

There is no specific antidote for OX toxicity, and treatment thus consists of general supportive and symptomatic measures.

3.4 MORANTEL

MO in many ways is similar to PY.

3.4.1 Action

The mode of action of MO is similar to that of PY. Its cholinergic activity has been measured via clamp techniques using cockroach motor neurones and using an antagonist, mecamylamine, to control the experiments [36]; importantly this experiment showed the striking difference between invertebrate acetylcholine receptors between insects and nematodes. MO and OX are both known to inhibit the enzyme fumarate reductase in parasitic worms as measured using the test system of *Helicobacter pylori* cell growth and viability; this study also found that OX was a greater inhibitor of this enzyme than MO [37]. There are, as with PY, differences in activity related to the salt form used; MO tartrate for example is more water-soluble than the parent compound MO. MO is administered in various forms: tartrate, fumarate, and citrate, and the pharmacodynamics of each salt is slightly different. MO is currently infrequently used in pets and is not used in human medicine, nor in general environmental activities, such as in crop pesticides or as a biocide.

3.4.2 Usage

Essentially MO has a low gastrointestinal absorption rate and is therefore a well-tolerated drug in horses and livestock. Cattle, for example, tolerate at least 10 times the therapeutic dose (which is 20 mg/kg) and can take up to 200 mg/kg. However care needs to be taken with calves, whose intestinal tracts are more absorptive in the early stages of life where intoxication can occur at 110 mg/kg. MO can cause fatalities in sheep with relatively low overdosing; the therapeutic dose here is between 7.5 and 15 mg/kg. Horses appear to be more susceptible than other domestic species and mild intoxication can occur at 70−80 mg/kg; here relatively mild symptoms can be seen, with moderate abdominal pain, tremors, dyspnoea, and ataxia occurring about 30 min after the administration of the drug, although these resolve within an hour. Care should always be taken when dosing with this drug in all individuals that have been fasting; the lack of food in the previous 24 h can induce serious intoxication and in some cases where doses are in the 80 mg/kg range this can cause death.

3.4.3 Safety and Toxicity

The signs of intoxication with MO involve the respiratory system more than they usually do with PR, although the intestinal presentation seen with the latter also occurs with MO. The signs of toxicity seen include dyspnea, tachypnea, hypersalivation, vomiting, and increased bowel activity, such as diarrhea and defecation. Neurological symptoms are also seen ranging from ataxia, tremors to convulsions. Severe adverse reactions are very rare at therapeutic doses with MO, nevertheless the drug should never be given to sick or weak individuals, and a damaged gastrointestinal mucosa can increase absorption and lead to toxicity. MO, like levamisole, is a nicotinic agent [38], and as they have similar actions it should not be administered with either PY or levamisole. Minerals are believed to reduce anthelminthic effectiveness of MO.

3.4.4 Species Differences

Little data exists that discusses in any detail differences between species in terms of safety issues or efficacy issues and further investigation is needed to fully explore this issue; however it is unlikely that major differences occur that are any different from those seen with other members of this group. Although MO is effective in sheep, for example, when given in combination with diethylcarbamazine [17], it should also be noted that resistance to MO has been reported in *H. contortus* in sheep [38]. The safety of MO in goats has also been demonstrated [39].

The tartrate of MO is very poorly absorbed into the bloodstream in ruminants, however the absorbed MO is quickly metabolized by the liver and is often not detected in plasma or in milk of lactating animals. Four days after oral administration less than 17% is excreted in the urine, as metabolites and 70% or more is lost in the feces as the unchanged parent molecule, thus the latter is the major source of excretion. It should be noted that MO breaks down quickly in feces, and appears to have neither insecticidal, bactericidal, nor fungicidal activity in these feces, and therefore the use of MO is thought not to compromise environmental integrity or be detrimental to the environment [29]. A hazard assessment of MO indicated that it is only a baseline toxicant when tested in a bioluminescence inhibition test with *Vibrio fisheri*, a test that measures bioavailability and uptake into biological membranes [40]; this study also showed that MO also has negligable effects on photosynthesis in green algae. MO therefore has less effect than ivermectin as an environmental hazard—ivermectin can pose an environmental problem for soil dwelling invertebrates in a way that MO does not—and thus the excreta from farm animals treated with MO are regarded as safe for the environment. This was shown in a study on soil invertebrates test organisms *Folsomia fimetaria* or *Enchytraeus cryptus* where MO was found not to induce significant mortality, even at high levels [41]. The tartrate is only slightly toxic to fish at levels greater than 40 µg/L and is toxic to carp and water fleas only at the same levels.

3.4.5 Contraindications

Organophosphates and diethylcarbamazine are both inhibitors of acetyl cholinesterase and therefore increase the toxicity when given with MO. In addition, MO and piperazines do have an effect of neutralizing each other through an antagonistic effect and therefore should never be given together. As with PR, the antidote for intoxication with MO is atropine. In terms of the use of MO in animals for consumption, the official allowable marker residue levels for MO (ie, the sum of residue that can be hydrolyzed to in animals for consumption—ie, for sheep and cattle) are as defined by authorities in the United States as $100\,\mu g/kg$ for muscle, $800\,\mu g/kg$ for liver, and $50\,\mu g/kg$ for milk [29].

3.5 DISCUSSION

These drugs have been useful contributors to veterinary and human medicine for a number of years, and currently still have value, particularly in combination with other anthelmintics such as the benzimidazoles and praziquantel. They are relatively safe as long as certain, relatively obvious precautions are taken, such as avoiding use with competing drugs, or those that might have a similar action and thus cause additive excessive effects.

Indeed the potential role of this drug group in contributing to the improvement of the efficacy of anthelmintic therapy in humans and animals could be argued to have not yet been completely fulfilled. In this current era of searching for new classes of drugs there is also the effort to repurpose existing drugs. It is quite possible, given the limited range of studies that have been carried out to date, that combinations of one of these three drugs with say benzimidazoles or compounds from other classes, such as emodepside, might be more efficacious against the difficult to treat parasites, such as *Trichuris* sp. and hookworms; the work mentioned above in Zanzibar [34] is encouraging.

From the perspective of safety, the subject of this chapter, this group appears on the whole to be very safe agents in mammals and for the environment, given that by their very nature of action all drugs do have the potential of carrying some negative effect or inherent consequences. That being said, the three drugs discussed here are not all equal in their safety profile, and in addition there are certainly restrictions with regard to the combination with other drugs that act on similar biological targets in the host and in the worms.

The use of drugs in humans and animals differs more in the experience and use that has been achieved to date than important differences between these two medicines. There is always more caution in the use of chemotherapeutic drugs for human use than in veterinary medicine, in part due to limitations in the ability to carry out drug detailed trials. As a consequence there are more restrictions placed on the use of these agents in humans at this point than there are in veterinary medicine. Most of the side effects of this group of drugs are as a result of their effect on the similar neurotransmission systems in the host and parasite rather than eliciting induced pathology or the effect of the death of the parasite targets—at least as far as intestinal worms are concerned and probably also with tissue parasites such as *Trichinella* sp. There are some differences in side reactions that are related to natural physiological differences in the host, such as age, but these are relatively limited. In addition there appear to be few safety issues related to repeated use of these agents and also no accumulative effect described.

Admittedly there is a fundamental difference in the approaches used by the veterinary and the human medical community with regards the purposing of anthelmintics, the former being more focused on reducing production costs and very high levels of efficacy to fit client needs, and the latter being more related to improving the overall health of those in developing countries (often carried out as humanitarian efforts by drug companies). Nevertheless, as happened in the past, there remains an important relationship between these two medical communities and the human medical world has always utilized to a great extent many veterinary drugs, a prime example that has been most successful is that seen with the macrolactone ivermectin.

It would seem that the possibility of combining one (or even perhaps two) of these three compounds together with other agents, such the powerful benzimidazole flubendazole, would be important pathways to take for further investigation. As highlighted in this discussion, an area of interest at present is addressing ways of improving the available treatments for *Trichuris* sp., particularly in the context of global programs aimed at controlling and eliminating intestinal helminths. However, the use of any of these drugs in mass administration programs in endemic areas adds a further degree of required safety, including the possibility of adverse reactions occurring due to the presence of coinfections with other parasites; such untoward events have happened with other mass programs such as the effect of hyper-loiasis on onchocerciasis mass treatment programs

[42]. Thus maintaining concern with the complete range of possibilities of adverse reactions when using a drug, or drugs, in the context of large endemic communities is essential.

In summary, the relatively safe profile of this group, the tetrahydropyrimidines, compared with other anthelmintics, and given the effectiveness of these agents (when used in anthelmintics combinations) on hardy parasites, suggest that this anthelmintic group should remain in contention as useful contributors to human and veterinary public health.

REFERENCES

[1] Austin WC, Courtney W, Danilewicz JC, Morgan DH, Conover LH, Howes HL, et al. Pyrantel tartrate, a new anthelmintic effective against infections of domestic animals. Nature 1966;212:1273—4.
[2] Martin RJ, Verma S, Levandoski M, Clark CL, Qian H, Stewart M, et al. Drug resistance and neurotransmitter receptors of nematodes: recent studies on the mode of action of levamisole. Parasitology 2005;131(Suppl):S71—84.
[3] Katz M. Anthelmintics. Drugs 1977;13:124—36.
[4] Atchison WD, Geary TG, Manning B, VandeWaa EA, Thompson DP. Comparative neuromuscular blocking actions of levamisole and pyrantel-type anthelmintics on rat and gastrointestinal nematode somatic muscle. Toxicol Appl Pharmacol 1992;112:133—43.
[5] Bapiro TE, Andersson TB, Otter C, Hasler JA, Masimirembwa CM. Cytochrome P450 1A1/2 induction by antiparasitic drugs: dose-dependent increase in ethoxyresorufin O-deethylase activity and mRNA caused by quinine, primaquine and albendazole in HepG2 cells. Eur J Clin Pharmacol 2002;58:537—42.
[6] Barski D, Spodniewska A. Activity of selected antioxidative enzymes in rats exposed to dimethoate and pyrantel tartrate. Pol J Vet Sci 2012;15:239—45.
[7] Beugnet F, Kerboeuf D, Nicolle JC, Soubieux D. Use of free living stages to study the effects of thiabendazole, levamisole, pyrantel and ivermectin on the fine structure of Haemonchus contortus and Heligmosomoides polygyrus. Vet Parasitol 1996;63:83—94.
[8] Mackenstedt U, Schmidt S, Mehlhorn H, Stoye M, Traeder W. Effects of pyrantel pamoate on adult and preadult Toxocara canis worms: an electron microscope and autoradiography study. Parasitol Res 1993;79:567—78.
[9] Cortinas de Nava C, Espinosa J, García L, Zapata AM, Martínez E. Mutagenicity of antiamebic and anthelmintic drugs in the Salmonella typhimurium microsomal test system. Mutat Res 1983;117:79—91.
[10] Otubanjo OA, Mosuro AA. An in vivo evaluation of induction of abnormal sperm morphology by some anthelmintic drugs in mice. Mutat Res 2001;497:131—8.
[11] Hennig UG, Galindo-Prince OC, Cortinas de Nava C, Savage EA, von Borstel RC. A comparison of the genetic activity of pyrvinium pamoate with that of several other anthelmintic drugs in Saccharomyces cerevisiae. Mutat Res 1987;187:79—89.
[12] Kotze AC, Stein PA, Dobson RJ. Investigation of intestinal nematode responses to naphthalophos and pyrantel using a larval development assay. Int J Parasitol 1999;29:1093—9.
[13] Ofori-Adjei D, Dodoo AA, Appiah-Danquah A, Couper M. A review of the safety of niclosamide, pyrantel, triclabendazole and oxamniquine. Int J Risk Safety Med 2008.

[14] DiPietro JA, Todd KS. Anthelmintics used in treatment of parasitic infections of horses. Vet Clin North Am Equine Pract 1987;3:1−14.

[15] Smith CF. Some aspects of the pharmacology of pyrantel. N Z Vet J 1973;21:52−3.

[16] Chartier C, Pors I, Benoit C. Efficacy of pyrantel tartrate against experimental infections with *Haemonchus contortus*, *Teladorsagia circumcincta* and *Trichostrongylus colubriformis* in goats. Vet Parasitol 1995;59:69−73.

[17] Cornwell RL. Controlled laboratory trials in sheep with the anthelmintic pyrantel tartrate. Vet Rec 1966;79:590−5.

[18] Fasanmade AA, Akanni AO, Olaniyi AA, Fasanmade AA, Tayo F. Bioequivalence of pyrantel pamoate dosage forms in healthy human subjects. Biopharm Drug Dispos 1994;15:527−34.

[19] Phuvanandh D, Dulyapiree Y, Chatisiri J, Panrong A, Tanskul P, Phuvanandh M. Efficacy of common broad spectrum anthelmintics against hook worm, *Ascaris* and *Trichiuris* in Hat Yai district, Songkhla Province, Thailand. J Med Assoc Thai 1994;77:357−62.

[20] Snow DH. The effects of pyrantel pamoate and tetrachlorethylene on several blood enzyme levels in the greyhound. Aust Vet J 1973;49:269−72.

[21] Spodniewska A, Zasadowski A. The effect of dimethoate and pyrantel on vitamin C concentration in the rat liver. Pol J Vet Sci 2006;9(1):23−9.

[22] Ferrara P, Bersani I, Bottaro G, Vitelli O, Liberatore P, Gatto A, et al. Massive proteinuria: a possible side effect of pyrantel pamoate? Ren Fail 2011;33:534−6.

[23] Okon ED. Effect of pyrantel tartrate on the third stage larvae of *Ascaridia galli*. Res Vet Sci 1976;21:104.

[24] Marchiondo AA, TerHune TN, Herrick RL. Target animal safety and tolerance study of pyrantel pamoate paste (19.13% w/w pyrantel base) administered orally to horses. Vet Ther 2005;6:311−24.

[25] Forbes LS. Toxicological and pharmacological relations between levamisole, pyrantel and diethylcarbamzine and their significance in helminth chemotherapy. Southeast Asian J Trop Med Publ Health 1972;3:235−41.

[26] Schmid K, Rohdich N, Zschiesche E, Kok DJ, Allan MJ. Efficacy, safety and palatability of a new broad-spectrum anthelmintic formulation in dogs. Vet Rec 2010;167:647−51.

[27] Hsu WH. Toxicity and drug interactions of levamisole. J Am Vet Med Assoc 1980;176:1166−9.

[28] Hsu WH. Drug interactions of levamisole with pyrantel tartrate and dichlorvos in pigs. Am J Vet Res 1981;42:1912−14.

[29] Fitzpatrick SC1, Vilim A, Lambert G, Yong MS, Brynes SD. Dietary intake estimates as a means to the harmonization of maximum residue levels for veterinary drugs. II. Proposed application to the Free Trade Agreement between the United States and Canada. Regul Toxicol Pharmacol 1996;24:177−83.

[30] Chapman MR, French DD, Monahan CM, Klei TR. Identification and characterization of a pyrantel pamoate resistant cyathostome population. Vet Parasitol 1996;66:205−12.

[31] Martin RJ, Robertson AP. Control of nematode parasites with agents acting on neuro-musculature systems: lessons for neuropeptide ligand discovery. Adv Exp Med Biol 2010;692:138−54.

[32] Martin RJ, Clark CL, Trailovic SM, Robertson AP. Oxantel is an N-type (methyridine and nicotine) agonist not an L-type (levamisole and pyrantel) agonist: classification of cholinergic anthelmintics in *Ascaris*. Int J Parasitol 2004;34:1083−90.

[33] Grandemange E, Fournel S, Boisramé B. Field evaluation of the efficacy and the safety of a combination of oxantel/pyrantel/praziquantel in the treatment of naturally acquired gastrointestinal nematode and/or cestode infestations in dogs in Europe. Vet Parasitol 2007;145:94−9.

[34] Speich B, Ali SM, Ame SM, Bogoch II, Alles R, Huwyler J, et al. Efficacy and safety of albendazole plus ivermectin, albendazole plus mebendazole, albendazole plus oxantel pamoate, and mebendazole alone against *Trichuris trichiura* and concomitant soil-transmitted helminth infections: a four-arm, randomised controlled trial. Lancet Infect Dis 2015;15:277−84.

[35] Speich B, Ame SM, Ali SM, Alles R, Huwyler J, Hattendorf J, et al. Oxantel pamoate-albendazole for *Trichuris trichiura* infection. N Engl J Med 2014;370:610−20.

[36] Pinnock RD, Sattelle DB, Gration KA, Harrow ID. Actions of potent cholinergic anthelmintics (morantel, pyrantel and levamisole) on an identified insect neurone reveal pharmacological differences between nematode and insect acetylcholine receptors. Neuropharmacology 1988;27:843−8.

[37] Mendz GL, Hazell SL, Srinivasan S. Fumarate reductase: a target for therapeutic intervention against *Helicobacter pylori*. Arch Biochem Biophys 1995;321:153−9.

[38] Yadav CL, Kumar R, Uppal RP, Verma SP. Multiple anthelmintic resistance in *Haemonchus contortus* on a sheep farm in India. Vet Parasitol 1995;60:355−60.

[39] Reinemeyer CR, Pringle JK. Evaluation of the efficacy and safety of morantel tartrate in domestic goats. Vet Hum Toxicol 1993;35(Suppl. 2):57−61.

[40] Escher BI, Berger C, Bramaz N, Kwon JH, Richter M, Tsinman O, et al. Membrane-water partitioning, membrane permeability, and baseline toxicity of the parasiticides ivermectin, albendazole, and morantel. Environ Toxicol Chem 2008;27:909−18.

[41] Jensen J, Diao X, Hansen AD. Single- and two-species tests to study effects of the anthelmintics ivermectin and morantel and the coccidiostatic monensin on soil invertebrates. Environ Toxicol Chem 2009;28:316−23.

[42] Boussinesq M, Gardon J, Gardon-Wendel N, Kamgno J, Ngoumou P, Chippaux JP. Three probable cases of *Loa loa* encephalopathy following ivermectin treatment for onchocerciasis. Am J Trop Med Hyg 1998;58:461−9.

CHAPTER 4

Formulations and Clinical Uses of Pyrimidine Compounds in Domestic Animals

C.R. Reinemeyer
East Tennessee Clinical Research, Inc., Rockwood, TN, United States

4.1 INTRODUCTION

The pyrimidine drug class has had a long and successful history of use for the treatment and control of nematode parasites in nearly all species of domestic mammals. Various compounds in this class have been developed commercially for use in dogs, cats, horses, swine, cattle, sheep, and goats. The pyrimidine class has gained wide acceptance due to its excellent safety profile, broad spectrum of activity against numerous common nematodes, and availability in multiple, and in some cases very novel, formulations. In recent years, pharmaceutical manufacturers have developed numerous broad spectrum, combination anthelmintics for use in dogs and cats, and the efficacy achieved by relatively low dosages of pyrimidines has made this class an ideal supplement for inclusion in such parasiticides. Even though pyrimidine resistance has been reported in several nematode species, as described in a separate chapter of this collection, many of these compounds continue to exhibit significant efficacy against important parasitic targets.

This presentation will present examples of the various pyrimidine formulations that have been approved for commercial distribution to veterinarians or consumers, and will discuss the anthelmintic properties and clinical applications of these compounds in domestic animals.

4.2 FORMULATIONS

Formulations are the physical forms in which a final medicinal product is administered to a patient. Examples of common formulations include solutions, suspensions, oral pastes, tablets, capsules, chewables, feed premixes, and topical products.

Pyrantel Parasiticide Therapy in Humans and Domestic Animals.
DOI: http://dx.doi.org/10.1016/B978-0-12-801449-3.00015-6
67

The following presentation is organized by individual pyrimidine compounds, with separate subcategories for each marketed formulation thereof. These are further subdivided by the domestic animal species for which products in that formulation have been registered. In some cases, multiple formulations of a given active ingredient have been developed for use in a single species. Concentrations of the active ingredients in the final formulation are presented, along with label indications of the respective pioneer product, when known, or those of a subsequent generic version.

The scope of coverage herein is limited to one representative product for each unique compound/formulation/species category that has received regulatory approval. Combination anthelmintics comprised of a pyrimidine plus one or more companion parasiticides are organized primarily by the number of active ingredients and secondarily by alphabetical order of non-pyrimidines listed on the product label. When two pyrimidine compounds are components of the same product, the representative formulation is listed under the active ingredient that is present in greater quantity. No attempt has been made to provide an exhaustive list of approved pioneer or generic products, and some formulations that are no longer commercially available have been included for the sake of completeness. The regulatory language cited herein largely reflects United States of America (USA) Food and Drug Administration/Center for Veterinary Medicine (FDA/CVM) standards, but exceptions are included for pyrimidine compounds or formulations that were never developed for veterinary use in the United States.

4.2.1 Pyrantel Pamoate

4.2.1.1 Suspension

A suspension is a dosing form in which insoluble or poorly soluble drugs are dispersed uniformly in a liquid medium by means of a suspending agent. Drugs in suspension often achieve greater bioavailability than other formulations intended for oral administration. Suspensions facilitate treatment of individual patients because accurate dosing can be achieved for animals of widely ranging body weights. With suspension formulations of pyrantel pamoate, the active agent may separate after storage, so it is always advisable to shake or stir the product thoroughly before preparing individual doses.

Suspension formulations of pyrantel pamoate have been approved for use in horses and dogs.

4.2.1.1.1 Equine

Strongid T (Zoetis); NADA 091–739, approved in the United States on October 19, 1973.

Oral suspension containing 50 mg pyrantel base as pyrantel pamoate per milliliter.

*For the removal and control of mature large strongyles (*Strongylus vulgaris, S. edentatus, S. equinus*); pinworms (*Oxyuris equi*); large roundworms (*Parascaris equorum*) and small strongyles in horses and ponies.*

4.2.1.1.2 Canine

Nemex, Nemex-2, RFD Liquid Wormer (Zoetis); NADA 100–237, approved in the United States on June 3, 1977.

Nemex: Oral suspension containing 2.27 mg pyrantel base as pyrantel pamoate per milliliter.

Nemex-2: Oral suspension containing 4.54 mg of pyrantel base as pyrantel pamoate per milliliter.

*For the removal of large roundworms (*Toxocara canis *and* Toxascaris leonina*) and hookworms (*Ancylostoma caninum *and* Uncinaria stenocephala*) in dogs and puppies. To prevent reinfestation of* Toxocara canis *in puppies and adult dogs and in lactating bitches after whelping.*

4.2.1.1.3 Feline

No pyrantel pamoate suspensions have been approved for use in cats in the United States, and none were found in the databases of Australian, Canadian, European Union, or New Zealand veterinary regulatory authorities.

4.2.1.2 Paste

Paste formulations are typically more concentrated than suspensions, but are similarly convenient for accurately dosing individual animals of variable body weights. Paste formulations of pyrantel pamoate have been approved for use in horses, cats and dogs.

4.2.1.2.1 Equine

Strongid Paste (Zoetis); NADA 129–831, approved in the United States on October 26, 1982.

A 19.13% oral paste containing 180 mg of pyrantel base as pyrantel pamoate per milliliter.

Pyrantel Pamoate Paste is indicated for the removal and control of mature infections of the following parasites:
    Large Strongyles: Strongylus vulgaris S. edentatus S. equinus; *Small Strongyles; Pinworms* Oxyuris equi; *Large Roundworms* Parascaris equorum.

Pyrantel Pamoate Paste (Phoenix Scientific Inc.); NADA 200-342, approved in the United States on April 18, 2005.

A 19.13% oral paste containing 7.2 g of pyrantel base in 37.6 g of paste.

For the removal and control of mature infections of large strongyles (Strongylus vulgaris, S. edentatus, S. equinus); *small strongyles; pinworms* (Oxyuris equi); *large roundworms* (Parascaris equorum) *and tapeworms* (Anoplocephala perfoliata) *in horses and ponies.*

For nematode parasites, administer as a single oral dose of 3 mg/lb. For tapeworms (*Anoplocephala perfoliata*), administer as a single oral dose of 6 mg/lb.

4.2.1.2.2 Feline

Anthel Plus Cat Wormer (Greyhorse Veterinary [N.Z.] Ltd.); Registration No. A003607; registered in New Zealand on October 7, 1991.

Oral paste containing 114.3 mg of pyrantel pamoate and 300 mg niclosamide per milliliter.

For the treatment of Roundworms (Toxascaris leonina, Toxocara cati), *and Tapeworms* (Dipylidium caninum), *in cats and kittens of all ages.*

4.2.1.2.3 Canine

Vitapet Wormaway Worming Paste for Dogs and Puppies (Masterpet Corporation Ltd.); Registration No. A007589, registered in Australia on June 2, 1999.

Oral paste containing pyrantel pamoate 30 mg/mL and niclosamide 200 mg/mL.

For control and treatment of Roundworm, Tapeworm, Hookworm (Toxocara canis, Toxascaris leonina, Dipylidium caninum, Taenia taeniaeformis, Ancylostoma caninum, and Uncinaria stenocephala).

4.2.1.3 Tablets and Chewables

Numerous tablet formulations containing pyrantel pamoate have been approved for use in dogs and cats, and the palatability of chewable formulations can greatly facilitate dosing by dog owners. The earliest tablets contained only pyrantel pamoate as the sole active ingredient. In contrast, the solid oral formulations developed more recently have generally combined pyrantel pamoate with one or more parasiticides in order to provide broad spectrum control of additional parasites such as heartworms, whipworms, tapeworms, or arthropods. Tablets and chewables are formulated as fixed dosing units that are labeled for treatment of specific weight ranges of animals; many products feature various sizes of tablets or chewables that contain incremental multiples of the active compounds. Accurate dosing of individual animals may require administration of multiple units from one or more weight ranges.

4.2.1.3.1 Canine

Nemex Tablets (Ralston Purina, Farnam); NADA 101-331, approved in the United States, November 14, 1978.

Tablets containing 22.7, 45.4 or 113.5 mg pyrantel base per tablet.

The dosage of pyrantel pamoate for small dogs (<5 lbs) is 10 mg/kg; larger dogs (>5 lbs) should be dosed at 5 mg pyrantel pamoate per kilogram of body weight.

For removal of ascarids (Toxocara canis; Toxascaris leonina) *and hookworms* (Ancylostoma caninum; Uncinaria stenocephala) *in dogs and puppies. To prevent reinfection of* T. canis *in puppies and adult dogs and in lactating bitches after whelping.*

Heartgard Plus; Heartgard Plus for Dogs (Merial); NADA 140-971, approved in the United States on January 15, 1993.

Heartgard Plus products are chewable tablets containing ivermectin and pyrantel pamoate, administered to provide a minimum dosage of 6 µg/kg ivermectin and 5 mg/kg pyrantel pamoate. Chewables are available in different sizes for various body weight ranges.

For use in dogs: Ivermectin [to prevent canine heartworm disease by eliminating the tissue larval stages of Dirofilaria immitis *for a month (30 days) after infection], and Pyrantel pamoate (for the treatment and control of adult* Toxocara canis, Toxascaris leonina, Ancylostoma caninum, Uncinaria stenocephala *and* Ancylostoma braziliense*).*

Virbantel; Sentry HC Worm X Plus (Virbac); NADA 141-261, approved in the United States on March 13, 2007.

Flavored chewables containing pyrantel pamoate and praziquantel. Chewables are dosed to provide a minimum dosage of 5 mg pyrantel pamoate and 5 mg praziquantel per kilogram body weight (2.27 mg pyrantel pamoate and 2.27 mg praziquantel per lb).

For the treatment and control of roundworms (Toxocara canis, Toxascaris leonina); hookworms (Ancylostoma caninum, Ancylostoma braziliense, Uncinaria stenocephala); and tapeworms (Dipylidium caninum, Taenia pisiformis) in dogs and puppies.

Drontal Plus Broad Spectrum Anthelmintic Tablets; Drontal Plus Tablets; Drontal Plus Taste Tabs (Bayer); NADA 141-007, approved in the United States on May 19, 1994.

Tablets containing praziquantel, pyrantel pamoate, and febantel. Tablets are sized to deliver 5—10 mg of praziquantel, 5—10 mg of pyrantel pamoate, and more than or equal to 25 mg of febantel per kilogram body weight.

Drontal™ Plus Broad Spectrum Anthelmintic Tablets are indicated for the removal of the following intestinal parasites in dogs: Tapeworms (Dipylidium caninum, Taenia pisiformis, Echinococcus granulosus, and Echinococcus multilocularis); hookworms (Ancylostoma caninum and Uncinaria stenocephala), ascarids (Toxocara canis, and Toxascaris leonina) and whipworms (Trichuris vulpis).

4.2.1.3.2 Feline

Pyran 35 (Pyrantel Tablets) (Vetoquinol N A Inc.); DIN 02184567, approved in Canada on October 25, 1996.

Tablet containing 35 mg pyrantel pamoate.

The recommended dosages of Pyran 35 for cats and dogs are 20 and 5 mg/kg, respectively.

Pyran 35 tablets are indicated for the treatment of the following parasite infestations in dogs, puppies and cats:
Cats: Roundworm (Toxocara cati); Hookworm (Ancylostoma spp.)
Dogs and Puppies: Roundworm (Toxocara canis; Toxascaris leonina); Hookworm (Ancylostoma caninum, Uncinaria stenocephala).

Drontal (Bayer Animal Health); NADA 141-008, approved in the United States on September 29, 1993.

Tablet containing 678.5 mg/g pyrantel pamoate and 58 mg/g praziquantel.

Drontal tablets are formulated to provide a minimum of 20 mg/kg pyrantel pamoate and 5—12.5 mg/kg praziquantel.

Drontal Tablets will remove Tapeworms (Dipylidium caninum, Taenia taeniaeformis), Hookworms (Ancylostoma tubaeforme) and Large Roundworms (Toxocara cati) in kittens and cats.

4.2.2 Pyrantel Embonate

Pyrantel embonate (European Pharmacopoeia) is considered to be synonymous with pyrantel pamoate (US Pharmacopeia). For some anthelmintics approved in New Zealand, pyrantel pamoate is listed in the registration details whereas the package label identifies the same chemical as pyrantel embonate. The label indications of these two pyrantel salts are virtually interchangeable at the same concentrations and dosages. Given this common identity, the only examples presented in this section are unique formulations or combination anthelmintics for which no comparable product containing pyrantel pamoate could be identified.

4.2.2.1 Suspension

4.2.2.1.1 Canine

Vets Choice for Puppies Worming Suspension (Bayer Australia Ltd Animal Health); Australian Pesticides and Veterinary Medicines Authority (APVMA) #80433, registered in Australia on May 7, 2015.

Suspension containing pyrantel embonate 14.4 mg/mL and febantel 15.0 mg/mL.

For the control of roundworms, hookworms and whipworms in puppies and small dogs. This product does not control tapeworms or heartworms.

4.2.2.2 Paste

4.2.2.2.1 Equine

Strategy-T Oral Broad Spectrum Worm Paste for Horses (Virbac [Australia] Pty Ltd); AVPMA #61370, registered in Australia on January 31, 2007.

Oral paste containing 260 mg/mL pyrantel embonate and 200 mg/mL oxfendazole.

The recommended therapeutic dosage is equivalent to 13 mg/kg pyrantel embonate and 10 mg/kg oxfendazole per kilogram body weight.

Treats and controls the following parasites: Large Strongyles: (Bloodworms) Strongylus spp., Triodontophorus spp. Small strongyles (cyathostomins): (Redworms) including benzimidazole resistant strains (adult and immature) Cyathostomum spp., Cylicocyclus spp., Cylicostephanus spp. Cylicodontophorus spp. Gyalocephalus spp. Large Roundworms: (Ascarids) Parascaris equorum (adult and immature) including ivermectin, moxidectin and abamectin resistant strains (Adult). Pinworms: (Seatworm) Oxyuris equi and also aids in the control of Tapeworm: Anoplocephala perfoliata.

Virbac Horse Wormer Oral Broad Spectrum Wormer and Boticide Paste for Horses; (Virbac [Australia] Pty. Limited); APVMA #57819; registered in Australia on March 7, 2005.

Oral paste containing ivermectin 5.3 mg/g, pyrantel embonate 345.1 mg/g, and praziquantel 39.8 mg/g.

For treatment and control of tapeworms and roundworms (including arterial larval stages of Strongylus vulgaris *and benzimidazole resistant small strongyles) bots, and skin lesions caused by summer sores and microfilariae.*

4.2.2.2.2 Feline

Aristopet Animal Health All Wormer Paste for Cats and Kittens (Aristopet Pty Ltd); AVPMA #49580, registered in Australia on March 14, 1997.

Oral paste containing pyrantel embonate 90 mg/g and niclosamide monohydrate 264 mg/g.

*For control of Roundworm (*Toxocara *spp. And* Toxascaris leonina*), Hookworm (*Ancylostoma *spp. and* Uncinaria stenocephala*) (also* A. braziliense *in NZ, Tapeworm (*Dipylidium caninum, Taenia *spp.) in cats.*

4.2.2.3 Tablets and Chewables

Literally dozens of pioneer and generic tablet or chewable formulations containing pyrantel embonate have been approved by regulatory agencies around the world. The only examples presented here are unique combination anthelmintics for which no comparable product containing pyrantel pamoate could be identified.

4.2.2.3.1 Canine

Fenpral Intestinal Wormer for Dogs (Arkolette Pty Ltd); AVPMA #56735, registered in Australia on September 9, 2003.

Tablet containing pyrantel embonate 14.0 mg, praziquantel 50.0 mg, and fenbendazole 250.0 mg.

*For the control of gastrointestinal worms in dogs including: Roundworm (*Toxocara canis, Toxascaris leonina*), Hookworm (*Ancylostoma caninum, Ancylostoma braziliense, Uncinaria stenocephala*), Whipworm (*Trichuris vulpis*), Hydatid tapeworm (*Echinococcus granulosus*), Common flea tapeworm (*Dipylidium caninum*),* Taenia *spp.*

4.2.2.3.2 Feline

Exelpet Ezy-Dose Intestinal All-Wormer for Cats (Exelpet Products a Div of Mars Australia Pty Ltd); AVPMA #53277, registered in Australia on February 28, 2001.

Oral bolus/chewable, each containing pyrantel embonate 292.5 mg and epsiprantel 13.4 mg.

> *For control of Roundworm* (Toxocara *spp.,* Toxascaris leonina*); Hookworm* (Ancylostoma *spp.,* Uncinaria stenocephala*); and Tapeworm* (Dipylidium caninum, Taenia *spp.).*

4.2.3 Pyrantel Tartrate

4.2.3.1 Type A Medicated Articles and Type C Medicated Feeds

Pyrantel tartrate apparently has been developed for veterinary applications only in North America. All finished formulations marketed are feed premixes (Type A) or pelleted products to be top-dressed or mixed in feed (Type C).

4.2.3.1.1 Equine

Strongid 48 (Zoetis); NADA 140-819, approved April 18, 1990.

Strongid 48 was originally formulated as a feed premix at a concentration of 10.6% (48 g/lb) as pyrantel tartrate. Subsequently, the feed premix was replaced by alfalfa-based, pelleted formulations containing pyrantel tartrate at 10.6 g/kg (eg, Strongid-C) or 21.1 g/kg (eg, Strongid-2X) to be top-dressed or mixed in feed. Pyrantel tartrate is used in a continuous feeding program at 2.64 mg/kg body weight daily. This product is unique among equine dewormers because its primary use is prophylactic rather than therapeutic.

> *For the prevention of* Strongylus vulgaris *larval infections in horses. For control of the following parasites in horses: LARGE STRONGYLES (adults)* S. vulgaris, S. edentatus; *SMALL STRONGYLES (adult and fourth-stage larvae)* Cyathostomum *spp.* Cylicocyclus *spp.,* Cylicostephanus *spp.,* Cylicodontophorus *spp.,* Poteriostomum *spp.,* Triodontophorus *spp., PINWORMS (adult and fourth-stage larvae)* Oxyuris equi *ASCARIDS (adult and fourth-stage larvae)* Parascaris equorum.

4.2.3.1.2 Porcine

Banminth 48 (Zoetis); Banminth Premix 80 (Zoetis); NADA 043-290, approved in the United States.

Type A Medicated Article; 10.6% (48 g/lb). Mixed to provide a complete feed containing pyrantel tartrate equivalent to 96 g/t (0.0106%) or 800 g/t (0.0881%).

Pyrantel tartrate can be administered to swine at different dosages, depending on whether the intended use is therapeutic (1 or 3 days) or prophylactic (continuous feeding program).

Treatment, single day regimen—A complete feed for therapeutic use should contain 800 g of pyrantel tartrate per ton (880 mg/kg) of feed. Treatment should be administered as a sole ration in an amount that will be consumed within a few hours. Overnight fasting improves consumption. For swine up to 200 lbs body weight, a dosage of 22 mg/kg should be administered as the sole ration. For swine more than 200 lbs, the standard dose is 2000 mg per animal.

For the removal and control of large roundworm (Ascaris suum) *and nodular worm* (Oesophagostomum) *infections of swine.*

Treatment, three day regimen—A complete feed for therapeutic use should contain 96 g of pyrantel tartrate per ton (106 mg/kg) of feed. Treatment should be administered as the sole ration for three consecutive days.

For treatment and control of large roundworm (Ascaris suum) *infections of swine.*

Prophylaxis—Premix is to be added to the ration so that the complete feed contains pyrantel tartrate equivalent to 96 g (0.0106%) per ton (106 mg/kg of feed). The complete feed should be offered continuously as the sole ration.

For aid in the prevention of migration and establishment of large roundworm (Ascaris suum) *infections; for aid in the prevention of establishment of nodular worm* (Oesophagostomum) *infections of swine.*

4.2.4 Pyrantel Citrate

4.2.4.1 Type B Medicated Feeds

4.2.4.1.1 Porcine

Pyrantel citrate apparently is no longer marketed anywhere in the world. Feed premix formulations of pyrantel citrate for swine were previously available in Europe, with a therapeutic dosage of 14 mg/kg. Several studies have determined that the citrate salt of pyrantel was suboptimal for use in swine. In controlled studies, putatively pyrantel-resistant strains of

Oesophagostomum dentatum were less susceptible to citrate than to pamoate salts [1]. Pyrantel pamoate/embonate is absorbed from the porcine gut to a lesser extent than citrate. Consequently, pamoate salts achieve higher drug concentrations in the ingesta of the hindgut of swine and provide greater efficacy against parasites of the large intestine [2].

4.2.5 Morantel Citrate

4.2.5.1 Paste

4.2.5.1.1 Ovine and Caprine

Oralject Goat and Sheep Wormer (Virbac [Australia] Pty Limited); APVMA # 38791, registered in Australia on July 23, 1986.

Oral paste containing morantel citrate 30 mg/mL.

For the control and treatment of morantel susceptible mature and immature roundworms of sheep and goats including strains resistant to benzimidazole chemicals: Barber's Pole Worm (Haemonchus contortus), Black Scour Worm (Trichostrongylus spp.), Small Brown Stomach Worm (Teladorsagia [Ostertagia] circumcincta), Stomach Hair Worm (Trichostrongylus axei), Small Intestinal Worm (Cooperia curticei), Thin Neck Intestinal Worm (Nematodirus spp.), Large Mouthed Bowel Worm (Chabertia ovina), Large Bowel Worm (Oesophagostomum venulosum).

4.2.5.2 Feed Premix (Oral Powder)

4.2.5.2.1 Porcine

Wormtec 30 Pig Wormer (Phibro Animal Health Pty Ltd); APVMA #37827, registered in Australia on June 30, 1988.

Feed premix containing 30 g morantel citrate per kilogram. Thoroughly mix 1 kg of Wormtec 30 with every ton of pig feed to be medicated. Administer continuously in the feed of pigs during the period for which roundworm and nodular worm control is required.

For the prevention of migration of roundworm (Ascaris suum) and the prevention of intestinal infections of roundworm (A. suum) and as an aid in the prevention of nodular worm (Oesophagostomum dentatum).

4.2.5.3 Oral Solution/Suspension

4.2.5.3.1 Porcine

Bomantel Water Soluble Wormer for Pigs (Bayer Australia Ltd. [Animal Health]); APVMA #59196, registered in Australia on December 22, 2005.

Oral solution/suspension containing 100 mg morantel citrate per milliliter.

In water additive for the prevention of migration of roundworm (Ascaris suum) and the prevention of intestinal infections of roundworm and as an aid in the prevention of nodular worm (Oesophagostomum dentatum).

4.2.6 Morantel Tartrate

Three formulations of morantel tartrate have been developed and approved for commercial use in the United States: a medicated feed pre-mix, oral boluses, and a novel, sustained release device for continuous administration of the active agent. In Australia and New Zealand, other formulations of morantel tartrate have been marketed for treatment of horses and swine.

4.2.6.1 Type A Medicated Article
4.2.6.1.1 Bovine
Rumatel 88 (Zoetis); NADA 092-444, approved in the United States on March 17, 1994.

Medicated premix containing 88 g of morantel tartrate per pound of product, and intended to be administered at a dosage of 10 mg/kg body weight. Morantel requires no milk withholding period, but cattle should not be slaughtered within 14 days of treatment.

For removal and control of mature gastrointestinal nematode infections of cattle including stomach worms (Haemonchus species, Ostertagia species, Trichostrongylus species), worms of the small intestine (Cooperia species, Trichostrongylus species, Nematodirus species), and worms of the large intestine (Oesophagostomum radiatum).

4.2.6.1.2 Caprine
Rumatel 88 (Zoetis); NADA 092-444, approved in the United States on March 17, 1994.

Type A medicated article containing 88 g of morantel tartrate per pound of product. Rumatel is used to produce a Type C medicated feed containing 0.44−4.4 g of morantel tartrate per pound. Complete feed is offered at 0.44 g of morantel tartrate per 100 lbs of body weight, providing a dosage of 10 mg/kg. When used at recommended levels, the slaughter withdrawal and milk discard periods for morantel tartrate in goats are 30 and 0 days, respectively.

For removal and control of mature gastrointestinal nematode infections of goats including Haemonchus contortus, Ostertagia (Teladorsagia) circumcincta, *and* Trichostrongylus axei.

4.2.6.1.3 Porcine
Banminth II (Phibro Animal Health Corporation); DIN 00327042, registered in Canada on December 31, 1977.

Feed premix containing 200 g of morantel tartrate per kilogram.

Mix to provide 1250 mg morantel tartrate per kilogram (0.125%) in complete feed.

Medicated feed is to be fed at the rate of 1 kg per 100 kg body weight. Optimal results are obtained by fasting animals overnight prior to treatment.

As an aid in the removal and control of gastrointestinal nematode infections of swine caused by the following parasites: Mature stomach worms (Hyostrongylus rubidus); *mature and immature large roundworms* (Ascaris suum); *mature and immature nodular worms* (Oesophagostomum *spp.).*

4.2.6.2 Bolus

4.2.6.2.1 Bovine
Nematel Cattle Wormer Bolus (Zoetis); NADA 093-903, approved in the United States on October 17, 1986.

Oral bolus containing 2.2 g of morantel tartrate equivalent to 1.3 g of morantel base. Product was dosed at 1 bolus per 500 lbs body weight (boluses could be divided in half for more accurate dosing) to provide 9.7 mg morantel tartrate per kilogram body weight. Nematel had milk and slaughter withdrawal periods of 0 and 14 days, respectively.

Use for the removal and control of mature gastrointestinal nematode infections of cattle, including stomach worms (Haemonchus *spp,* Ostertagia *spp, and* Trichostrongylus *spp), worms of the small intestine* (Cooperia *spp,* Trichostrongylus *spp,* Nematodirus *spp), and worms of the large intestine* (Oesophagostomum radiatum).

4.2.6.3 Sustained Release Device

4.2.6.3.1 Bovine
Paratect Cartridge (Zoetis); NADA 134-779, approved in the United States on December 7, 1984.

Sustained-release bolus providing 11.8 mg morantel base per animal, and dosed at one bolus per calf (≥200 lbs body weight). The Paratect

Cartridge was a reservoir system designed to provide constant delivery of morantel tartrate for an entire grazing season after a single dosing event. The Paratect Cartridge consisted of a stainless steel cylinder (2.5 cm diameter × 10 cm length) with porous polyethylene disks at either end that were impregnated with cellulose triacetate. The reservoir within the cartridge was filled with a mixture of morantel tartrate and polyethylene glycol [3]. After deposition within the rumen, drug diffused through the membranes and provided continuous therapeutic concentrations of morantel tartrate for approximately 90 days.

For control of the adult stage of the following gastrointestinal nematode infections in weaned calves (≥200 lbs) and yearling cattle: Ostertagia spp., Trichostrongylus axei, Cooperia spp., and Oesophagostomum radiatum. Efficacy is dependent upon continuous control of the gastrointestinal parasites for approximately 90 days following administration.

Paratect Flex Diffuser (Zoetis); NADA 134-779, approved in the United States on 25 March, 1991.

The Paratect Flex Diffuser consisted of an extruded sheet containing drug and ethylene vinyl acetate (EVA) sandwiched between thin films of EVA; a symmetrical pattern of circular perforations was punched through the sheet. Drug release occurred from the uncoated edges of the central lamina. The trilaminated sheet was formed into a cylinder, with plastic plugs in both ends. The core lamina contained 19.8 g of morantel tartrate equivalent to 11.8 g of morantel base. The Paratect Flex was administered orally, using a special dosing gun. The device was retained in the rumen and morantel was released continuously for approximately 90 days.

For control of the adult stage of the following gastrointestinal nematode infections in weaned calves (≥200 lbs) and yearling cattle: Ostertagia spp., Trichostrongylus axei, Cooperia spp., and Oesophagostomum radiatum. Efficacy is dependent upon continuous control of the gastrointestinal parasites for approximately 90 days following administration.

4.2.6.4 Paste
4.2.6.4.1 Equine
Equiban Paste (Zoetis Australia Pty Ltd); APVMA #50080, registered in Australia on July 30, 1997.

Oral paste containing 150 mg of morantel tartrate per gram.

For the control of large strongyles (Strongylus spp.), small strongyles (Cyathostomes), large roundworm (Parascaris equorum) and pinworm

(Oxyuris equi) in horses. Good activity has been demonstrated against tapeworm (Anoplocephala perfoliata*), and lumen dwelling immature forms of* Cyathostomum *spp.,* Triodontophorus *spp. and* Strongylus vulgaris*.*

Ammo Allwormer Paste for Horses (Ceva Animal Health (NZ) Ltd); AVPMA #A009601, registered in New Zealand on January 25, 2006.

Oral paste containing morantel tartrate 167 mg and abamectin 4 mg/g.

Administer at 0.2 mg/kg abamectin and 8.35 mg/kg morantel tartrate.

Controls the following parasites of horses: Tapeworms: Anoplocephala perfoliata*. Large Strongyles:* Strongylus vulgaris *(adults and arterial larval stages),* Strongylus edentatus *(adult and tissue stages),* Strongylus equinus *(adults) and* Triodontophorus *spp. (adults). Small Strongyles: Including benzimidazole resistant strains of adult and immature:* Cyathostomum *spp.,* Cylicocyclus *spp.,* Cylicostephanus *spp.,* Cylicodontophorus *spp.,* Gyalocephalus *sp. Pinworms:* Oxyuris equi *(adult and immature). Ascarids:* Parascaris equorum *(adult and immature). Hairworms:* Trichostrongylus axei *(adult). Large Mouth Stomach Worms:* Habronema muscae *(adult). Bots:* Gasterophilus *spp. (oral and gastric stages). Lungworms:* Dictyocaulus arnfieldi *(adult and immature). Intestinal Threadworms:* Strongyloides westeri *(adult). Also effective for the control of skin lesions caused by* Habronema*.*

Moranox Broadspectrum Oral Worming Paste for Horses (Arkolette Pty Ltd T/A Riverside Veterinary Products); APVMA #63652, registered in Australia on July 4, 2014.

Oral paste containing 245 mg morantel tartrate and 175 mg oxfendazole per gram. Administer paste at 10 mg/kg oxfendazole and 14 mg/kg morantel tartrate.

Used for the treatment and control of susceptible stains of small strongyles (including arterial larval stages of Strongylus vulgaris *and benzimidazole resistant small strongyles.*

4.2.6.5 Oral Granules, Pellets
4.2.6.5.1 Equine
Equiban granules (Zoetis Australia Pty Ltd.); APVMA #49805, registered in Australia on April 2, 1997.

Oral granules, pellets containing 115 mg morantel tartrate per gram. Dose at 10 mg morantel tartrate per kilogram body weight.

*For the control of large strongyles (*Strongylus *spp.), small strongyles (Cyathostomes), large roundworm (*Parascaris equorum*) and pinworm (*Oxyuris equi*) in horses. Good activity has been demonstrated against tapeworm*

(Anoplocephala perfoliata) *and lumen dwelling immature forms of* Cyathostomum *spp.,* Triodontophorus *spp. and* Strongylus vulgaris.

4.2.7 Oxantel Pamoate/Embonate

Anthelmintic treatment of dogs is the sole application of oxantel salts in veterinary medicine, and the spectrum of activity appears to be limited to canine whipworms (*Trichuris vulpis*). The unique efficacy of oxantel against whipworms may be due to differences in the dominant cholinergic receptor subtype present in *Trichuris* compared to other nematodes [4]. In order to provide a wider spectrum of activity against common nematode parasites, oxantel is invariably coupled with pyrantel pamoate/embonate. Standard label indications for such combinations include removal or treatment of roundworms or ascarids (*Toxocara canis, Toxascaris leonina*) and hookworms (*Ancylostoma caninum, Uncinaria stenocephala*) through the action of pyrantel pamoate/embonate, and treatment of whipworms courtesy of oxantel salts.

Numerous products containing oxantel pamoate/embonate have been approved in Australia, Canada, and New Zealand. Table 4.1 presents basic descriptive information for one example of each unique formulation or anthelmintic combination containing oxantel pamoate or oxantel embonate.

4.3 CLINICAL USES OF PYRIMIDINE COMPOUNDS IN DOMESTIC ANIMALS

The terminology used in anthelmintic label indications reflects guidelines which are written and interpreted by the governing regulatory agencies. In the United States, those responsibilities are administered by the FDA/CVM. In the European Union, Australia, Canada, and New Zealand, the controlling regulatory bodies are the European Medicines Agency, Australian Pesticides and Veterinary Medicines Agency, Veterinary Drugs Directorate of Health Canada, and the ministry for Agricultural Compounds and Veterinary Medicines, respectively.

The FDA/CVM employs four distinct terms to indicate relative differences in efficacy and potential clinical uses of anthelmintics [5]. Products labeled by the FDA/CVM for "treatment" or "removal" are expected to eliminate more than or equal to 90% of a target parasite population, and are intended to be used therapeutically to ameliorate current or potential

Table 4.1 Canine anthelmintic formulations containing oxantel pamoate/embonate

Formulation	Brand name (Mfr), [country], registration no.	Oxantel salt, concentration	Active ingredient #2, concentration	Additional active ingredients, concentration	Unique indications[a]
Tablet	Pyr-A-Pam Plus Tablets (Zoetis Canada Inc), [Canada], DIN #00421464	Oxantel pamoate, 140 mg/tablet	Pyrantel pamoate, 35 mg/tablet	None	None
Tablet	Paratak Plus (Bayer New Zealand Ltd), [New Zealand], #A6456	Oxantel pamoate 545 mg/tablet	Pyrantel pamoate, 140 mg/tablet	Praziquantel, 50 mg/tablet	*Echinococcus granulosus*, *Taenia* spp., *Dipylidium caninum*
Tablet	Popantel Allwormer Plus Heartworm Tablets (Jurox Pty Ltd), [Australia], #54678	Oxantel embonate, 1084 mg/tablet	Ivermectin, 120 µg/tablet	Pyrantel embonate, 286 mg/tablet and Praziquantel, 100 mg/tablet	*Dirofilaria immitis*, *Echinococcus granulosus*, *Taenia pisiformis*, *Taenia ovis*, *Taenia hydatigena*, *Dipylidium caninum*
Chewable	Guardian Complete Worming Chew Monthly Heartworm and Intestinal Allwormer for Dogs (Intervet Australia Pty Ltd), [Australia], #58819	Oxantel embonate, 543 mg/chew	Ivermectin, 60 µg/chew	Pyrantel embonate, 143 mg/chew and Praziquantel, 50 mg/chew	*Ancylostoma braziliense*, *Ancylostoma ceylanicum*, *Dirofilaria immitis*, *Echinococcus granulosus*, *Taenia pisiformis*, *Taenia ovis*, *Taenia hydatigena*, *Dipylidium caninum*

[a]In addition to the usual spectrum for dogs (ie, ascarids, hookworms, and whipworms).

disease conditions. Products labeled for "control" may be somewhat less effective, but it is anticipated that repeated administration or persistent activity will reduce reinfection of the host. Products labeled for "prevention" are expected to inhibit the establishment of an adult worm population when administered prior to exposure to the infective stage.

This regulatory language addresses the most common circumstances in which anthelmintics would be used in clinical practice. Each option is relevant because the medical justifications for deworming can vary widely, even for the same drug against a specific parasitism. For example, a labeled anthelmintic would be used "therapeutically" when clinical signs are consistent with a specific parasitism (eg, anemia with hookworm infection). In companion animal practice, however, it is probably more common to dispense the same therapeutic anthelmintic for individual animals on the basis of a fecal diagnostic result, regardless of whether clinical disease is evident. One could argue whether such "empirical/therapeutic" doses are warranted for a healthy animal, but a positive diagnostic result indicates that the patient resides in a contaminated environment, and many of the common nematode parasites of dogs and cats have important zoonotic potential. Another common approach is to administer anthelmintics repeatedly to remove recurring helminth infections and to reduce environmental contamination with reproductive products. This practice embodies the pharmaceutical industry's rationale for adding therapeutic anthelmintics to heartworm preventives. Monthly administration of such combinations not only precludes establishment of *Dirofilaria* infections, but simultaneously accomplishes "control" of other common nematodes.

From a therapeutic standpoint, pyrimidines would be classified as broad spectrum anthelmintics because they are effective against helminths in two or more nematode superfamilies (eg, Strongyloidea and Ascaridoidea). A consistent feature of broad spectrum anthelmintic performance is that one helminth species is affected to a markedly lesser degree than other susceptible species after exposure to the same dosage. These organisms are termed "dose-limiting species" or "dose-limiting parasites."

Dose-limiting species present important issues for regulatory consideration. For example, the recommended use level of a marketed anthelmintic is determined de facto by the dosage required to achieve the minimum regulatory standard for a label indication against the dose-limiting parasite. Consequently, other labeled helminth targets are often susceptible to dosages that are substantially lower than the label stipulation. Another regulatory consideration for a dose-limiting species is that it will be designated as the preferred target in studies attempting to demonstrate the bioequivalence of a generic anthelmintic through biological endpoint comparisons. Similarly, noninterference studies with combination anthelmintics typically do not require evaluation of efficacy against all target species covered by label indications, but rather focus on the dose-limiting species of each component drug.

Numerous generic versions of pyrimidine compounds have been developed and marketed over the years, most notably generic formulations of pyrantel pamoate/embonate. Regulatory guidelines require that generic versions of any veterinary drug must list the same label claims as the "pioneer" compound, which is defined as the first product approved for commercial distribution that contained the active agent in the same concentration, formulation, and for the same intended uses. Substantial differences from the pioneer product in dosages, formulations, route of administration, label claims, or manufacturing processes that might affect drug bioavailability would require separate regulatory consideration for the generic candidate.

The following presentation will discuss clinical uses of pyrimidines in domestic animals. These discussions are organized by host species, target parasite(s), and pyrimidine compounds that are labeled for use in that host– parasite system. Examples of therapeutic, control, and/or preventive uses will be cited when applicable, and special regimens for specific parasitic conditions will be described.

4.3.1 Clinical Uses of Pyrimidines in Dogs

Pyrantel pamoate/embonate
Oxantel pamoate/embonate

4.3.1.1 Hookworms

Canine hookworms include *Ancylostoma caninum, A. braziliense,* and *Uncinaria stenocephala*. Hookworm infection is one of the most common diagnoses in canine practice, and *A. caninum* is by far the most prevalent species involved. *Ancylostoma* eggs were identified in 19% of canine fecal samples collected from various locales in the United States [6].

Ancylostoma caninum infections can be acquired by vertical (transmammary) transmission, percutaneous invasion, or ingestion of infective third-stage larvae or paratenic hosts. In mature dogs with some acquired immunity, infective larvae may not develop directly into adults, but rather migrate to somatic tissues such as kidney and skeletal muscle, where they undergo prolonged arrested development [7]. These arrested larvae are most commonly reactivated by the hormones of pregnancy and lactation, and larvae are transmitted to suckling pups in the bitch's milk. Although hookworm infection is observed in dogs of all ages, pups and juveniles are more likely to exhibit clinical signs of disease, including anemia, weakness, melena, anorexia, and weight loss or poor growth. As with most parasitisms, clinical signs are exacerbated by malnutrition, stress, or concurrent disease.

Hookworm disease (ancylostomosis) has been classified as four distinct syndromes which vary with the age, route of infection, or overall health status of the animal. In *peracute* ancylostomosis, suckling pups around 2—3 weeks of age die of severe anemia with no preceding clinical signs, due to overwhelming hookworm infections acquired through the transmammary route. *Acute* ancylostomosis involves slightly older or weaned pups that survive long enough to develop melena and signs of severe anemia. Again, transmammary infection is the usual route. The two remaining classifications of ancylostomosis occur in mature dogs that are either repeatedly exposed to L3 stages or are continuously reinfected with larvae activated from their arrested, somatic pools. *Uncompensated* ancylostomosis occurs when malnutrition or co-morbid disease render an animal incapable of managing hookworm insults through immunologic or general defense mechanisms. In contrast, no clinical signs are seen in dogs with *compensated* ancylostomosis, which is a term used to describe recurrent infections that are partially controlled, but not eliminated, by host mechanisms. Compensated ancylostomosis is typically recognized when fecal examinations after repeated treatments document the incessant reappearance of hookworm eggs.

Products labeled for treatment or removal of *Ancylostoma caninum* are the appropriate therapeutic choice for apparently healthy dogs or those with moderate signs of ancylostomosis (ie, compensated and uncompensated cases). Suckling pups with acute ancylostomosis require immediate and vigorous medical attention. Pyrantel pamoate/embonate is the preferred anthelmintic for this syndrome, due to its speed of activity and broad safety in debilitated animals. Ancillary medical management (eg, iron supplementation) is critical, but pups with acute ancylostomosis often make very dramatic recoveries once the immediate source of blood loss has been eliminated. By definition, anthelmintic treatment would arrive too late to salvage pups with peracute ancylostomosis, but surviving littermates should be treated promptly as for the acute syndrome.

Specific regimens of pyrantel pamoate have been designed to reduce the clinical impact of hookworm infections in suckling pups. These are described in greater detail in the section on *Toxocara canis*.

Current standards of care support the maintenance of all canine patients on some form of heartworm prevention, and all currently marketed *Dirofilaria* preventives are anthelmintics of the macrocyclic lactone (ML) class. Several heartworm preventive products have been developed in which the ML component is combined with other anthelmintics, including pyrimidines, to provide a broader spectrum of nematode control. Because most MLs also exhibit activity against hookworms, some of these combination products achieve higher efficacy against hookworms than either component used singly. For example, HeartGard Plus (ivermectin plus pyrantel pamoate) was more than 99% effective against adult *Uncinaria stenocephala* whereas pyrantel pamoate alone exhibited 93.4—96.3% efficacy [8]. Regular, monthly administration of such combination products reduces environmental contamination with hookworm eggs, and thereby reduces the risk of compensated or uncompensated ancylostomosis in mature dogs.

Uncinaria stenocephala is a less common hookworm of dogs that is most often acquired through ingestion of third-stage larvae (L3s). *Uncinaria* is more restricted in its geographic distribution than *Ancylostoma caninum*, occurring more frequently in Europe, Canada, and the northern tier of the United States. *Uncinaria* eggs were found in only 1.02% of canine fecal samples collected from around the United States [6]. *Uncinaria* ingests plasma proteins rather than whole blood, so clinical signs are primarily related to the gradual loss of vital nutrients. *Ancylostoma braziliense* is another fairly nonpathogenic hookworm of dogs that is limited to tropical and subtropical climates.

Routine *Uncinaria* and *A. braziliense* infections can be managed with approved anthelmintics containing pyrantel pamoate/embonate. Transmammary transmission does not occur with either species, so special regimens for suckling pups are not required. Some monthly heartworm preventives are also labeled for efficacy against *U. stenocephala* and *A. braziliense* (eg, HeartGard Plus). Regular control is advisable in endemic areas because both *U. stenocephala* and *A. braziliense* can cause a zoonotic condition known as cutaneous *larva migrans* [9].

4.3.1.2 Ascarids

The ascarids or roundworms infecting dogs include *Toxocara canis* and less commonly, *Toxascaris leonina* and *Baylisascaris procyonis*. *Toxocara* infections are extremely common in suckling and weaned pups up to approximately 6 months of age. *Toxocara canis* eggs were found in more than 30% of canine fecal samples examined from various sources in the United States [6]. Patent infections are observed occasionally in mature dogs, but the associated worm numbers are usually modest.

Toxocara infections can be acquired by vertical (prenatal) transmission, or by ingestion of larvated eggs or paratenic hosts. Like hookworms in mature dogs, exposure of immune hosts to ascarid infection generally results in arrested larvae accumulating in somatic pools rather than adult worms establishing in the small intestine [10]. In bitches, pregnancy reactivates arrested *Toxocara* larvae which migrate into fetal pups prior to birth. Newborn pups generally develop patent infections by the third week of life. Clinical signs of disease include anorexia, diarrhea, weight loss or poor growth, ill thrift, respiratory signs, and a pot-bellied appearance. Clinical signs are more severe when accompanied by malnutrition, stress, or concurrent disease.

Toxocara canis is the dose-limiting parasite for pyrantel compounds in dogs. Pyrantel pamoate/embonate is used frequently to treat patent ascarid infections, but pyrimidines are only active against life cycle stages within the lumen of the gut. Accordingly, it is common practice to administer a second therapeutic dose approximately 2 weeks after the first, to remove worms that were immature or migrating through somatic tissues at the time of the first treatment.

Specific regimens of pyrantel pamoate/embonate have been prescribed to reduce ascarid burdens in suckling pups, and also to prevent environmental contamination with *Toxocara* eggs. It is commonly recommended that puppies be treated at 2, 4, 6, and 8 weeks of age with approved, therapeutic anthelmintics [11], and some authorities recommend various modifications of this basic schedule. Lactating bitches should be treated at the same intervals as their pups, as they also may develop patent infections after whelping. When a broad spectrum anthelmintic such as pyrantel pamoate/embonate is used, this same regimen provides excellent control of *Ancylostoma caninum* infections acquired by the transmammary route.

Although a program of intensive, repeated deworming greatly improves the health and viability of suckling pups, an equally important objective is to prevent environmental contamination with ascarid and hookworm eggs. Both of these reproductive products are potential sources of important zoonotic diseases. Humans who inadvertently ingest infective *Toxocara* eggs may develop visceral *larva migrans* or ocular *larva migrans* [12], and cutaneous *larva migrans* can result when human skin is invaded by third-stage hookworm larvae [9].

For older dogs, repeated monthly treatments in the form of a combination heartworm preventive effectively reduce environmental contamination with *T. canis* eggs.

Toxascaris leonina is an uncommon ascarid that is transmitted by ingestion of infective eggs or paratenic hosts. This roundworm species does not migrate systemically in dogs or cats, and thus cannot be transmitted vertically. For the same reason, *Toxascaris* does not cause zoonotic infections. Virtually all pyrantel formulations approved for use in dogs have label claims for efficacy against *Toxascaris*.

Baylisascaris procyonis is a very common ascarid of raccoons, but dogs that become infected by ingestion of larvated eggs or paratenic hosts may pass viable eggs in their feces. Inadvertent human ingestion of larvated *Baylisascaris* eggs can result in serious disease involving larval migration within the central nervous system [13]. Although no veterinary anthelmintics are currently labeled for adult *Baylisascaris* infections in dogs, most products with activity against canine ascarids, including pyrantel compounds, also exhibit some efficacy against *Baylisascaris*. Monthly administration of combination heartworm preventives that are labeled for *Toxocara* is recommended for any dog that has been diagnosed with a prior *Baylisascaris* infection [14].

4.3.1.3 Whipworms

The canine whipworm, *Trichuris vulpis*, is a fairly common parasite of adult dogs. *Trichuris* eggs were identified in 14.3% of fecal samples collected from shelter dogs and in 10% of dogs presented to veterinary hospitals [6].

Trichuris infections are acquired only through ingestion of larvated eggs, which can survive for several months in the environment. The prepatent period of canine whipworms is approximately 10−15 weeks, so infections are never observed in suckling pups. *Trichuris vulpis* is a more frequent cause of alimentary disease than any other helminth parasite of mature dogs. Clinical signs include those of large bowel diarrhea, weight loss, and ill-thrift.

Pyrantel pamoate/embonate exhibits little therapeutic activity against *Trichuris vulpis* in dogs. Nevertheless, several combination anthelmintics containing pyrantel pamoate/embonate are labeled for efficacy against whipworms, but any trichuricidal activity is invariably supplied by one of the alternate components. A relevant example is Drontal Plus (pyrantel pamoate + praziquantel + febantel). In a study with 25 dogs harboring naturally acquired whipworm infections, pyrantel pamoate alone or combined with praziquantel exhibited 0% efficacy against *Trichuris*. The addition of febantel to the latter combination, however, provided 93.9% efficacy against whipworms [15].

Oxantel, either alone or in combination with pyrantel pamoate/embonate, is the only pyrimidine compound with apparent activity against *Trichuris*. In Australia and New Zealand, oxantel plus pyrantel have been combined with ivermectin and/or praziquantel to provide products with a broader spectrum of activity against common helminths (Table 4.1).

4.3.1.4 Miscellaneous Canine Nematodes

Although no specific label claims have been filed, pyrantel pamoate apparently has some efficacy against *Physaloptera* spp. in dogs. Treatment of one naturally infected dog with 5 mg/kg pyrantel pamoate resulted in expulsion of mature worms that were identified as *Physaloptera rara* [16]. Several dogs with chronic vomiting had endoscopically confirmed *Physaloptera* infections. Mechanical removal combined with pyrantel pamoate treatment resolved clinical signs in all dogs available for follow-up [17].

4.3.2 Clinical Uses of Pyrimidines in Cats

Pyrantel Pamoate/Embonate

4.3.2.1 Ascarids

Toxocara cati is the most common nematode of domestic felids, with prevalences exceeding 25% in cats from some locales [18].

Cats acquire *T. cati* infections via the transmammary route, or by ingesting larvated eggs or paratenic hosts [10]. When *T. cati* is acquired through predation, the larvae are not exposed to the cat's immune effectors. Thus, recurrent ascarid infections are very common in mature cats that are competent hunters. *Toxocara cati* is not very pathogenic, and clinical signs of infection, if any, are usually limited to diarrhea, vomiting, weight loss or poor growth, rough hair coat, and abdominal enlargement.

Toxocara cati is the dose-limiting species for pyrantel pamoate in cats, and a dosage of 20 mg/kg was required to achieve more than or equal to 90% removal of ascarids [19]. It is interesting that this dosage is four times higher than that required for ascarids in dogs, whereas 5 mg/kg was effective against *T. leonina* in both host species.

Toxocara cati has some zoonotic potential as a potential agent of visceral or ocular *larva migrans*, so elimination of environmental contamination with infective eggs is desirable. To that end, some cat breeders treat new litters and nursing queens with pyrantel pamoate or another approved dewormer at various intervals after birth.

Several combination anthelmintics comprised of pyrantel pamoate/ embonate plus another active agent have been developed for feline use. In all cases, the supplemental dewormers (ie, epsiprantel, niclosamide, or praziquantel) were included to add cestodes to the spectrum of activity.

Dissimilar to common management practices for dogs, repeated anthelmintic treatment of cats at regular intervals is rarely employed as a control measure. This may be partially attributable to the absence of approved heartworm preventives for cats that include pyrantel pamoate. Although outdoor or predatory cats will almost certainly experience recurrent ascarid infections, treatment is usually based on the results of a recent fecal examination.

Toxascaris leonina also occurs in cats. The only routes of infection are ingestion of larvated eggs or paratenic hosts; vertical transmission is unknown. Treatment decisions are based on a positive fecal diagnosis.

4.3.2.2 Hookworms

The hookworms of cats include *Ancylostoma tubaeforme* and *A. braziliense*. Hookworm infection is not common in most feline populations, with prevalences ranging from 1% to 20% in fecal surveys [20].

Ancylostoma tubaeforme infections can be acquired by ingestion of infective third-stage larvae or paratenic hosts [7]. This species is not capable of percutaneous infection, and vertical transmission does not occur. Although hookworm infection is observed in cats of all ages, clinical signs are more common in kittens, and include slight anemia, weakness, melena, anorexia, and weight loss or poor growth. *Ancylostoma braziliense* occurs in both dogs and cats in warmer climates, but it rarely causes clinical signs.

Ancylostoma braziliense is the most common cause of cutaneous *larva migrans* in humans [9], so zoonotic considerations support more rigorous control of feline hookworm infections in warmer climates.

Hookworm infections of individual cats can be managed in much the same manner as *T. cati*. The absence of vertical transmission by either

A. tubaeforme or *A. braziliense* reduces the need for repeated treatments of suckling kittens raised under conditions of reasonable hygiene.

4.3.2.3 Miscellaneous Feline Nematodes

No pyrimidine products are labeled for use against *Physaloptera* spp. infections in cats or dogs. Repeated treatment of a single cat with pyrantel pamoate (5 mg/kg; two doses 3 weeks apart) was reportedly effective against *Physaloptera* spp. [21].

4.3.3 Clinical Uses of Pyrimidines in Horses

> *Pyrantel pamoate/embonate*
> *Pyrantel tartrate*
> *Morantel tartrate*

4.3.3.1 Large Strongyles (Strongylinae)

The most commonly cited distinction between large strongyles (ie, *Strongylus* spp.) and the so-called small strongyles is that only the former undergo systemic migration during development within the host. As adults, large strongyles are found attached to the mucosal surfaces of the cecum and colon.

Strongylus vulgaris is commonly offered as the model for a typical large strongyle life cycle. Horses acquire *S. vulgaris* by ingesting infective third-stage larvae from the environment while grazing. Larvae penetrate the intestinal wall and migrate within local arteries until the majority congregate at one common site, the root of the cranial mesenteric artery (CMA). These stages induce lesions of severe local arteritis, commonly referred to as "verminous aneurysms." Larval arteritis is considered to be a major cause of colic in the horse. After residing in the CMA for approximately 3 months, fourth-stage *S. vulgaris* larvae return to the wall of the large intestine and complete development to the adult stage. Ultimately, these new arrivals emerge into the lumen of the gut and begin to produce eggs approximately 6 months after the initial infection.

Other *Strongylus* species, *S. edentatus* and *S. equinus*, undergo similar migrations through other visceral tissues, and have prepatent periods of approximately 11 and 8 months, respectively.

4.3.3.1.1 Pyrantel Pamoate/Embonate for Treatment of Large Strongyles

In some of the earliest evaluations of pyrantel pamoate as a candidate dewormer for horses, single doses of pyrantel pamoate (7.2 or 6.6 mg/kg via nasogastric tube, or 6.6 mg/kg in feed) were 98%, 98%, and 99% effective, respectively, against adult *S. vulgaris* [22]. The same respective dosages and routes were also 89%, 62%, and 66% effective against *S. edentatus*, which is considered to be the dose-limiting species for pyrantel pamoate in horses. These studies also documented good efficacy against other, nonmigratory large strongyles, including *Oesophagodontus robustus* and four species of the genus *Triodontophorus*.

Because arterial larvae are the most pathogenic stage of the *S. vulgaris* life cycle, they have been investigated intensively as a potential target of anthelmintic treatment or immunologic manipulation [23]. However, pyrantel salts have no efficacy against these larval stages, presumably because pyrimidines are not absorbed systemically to any appreciable extent.

4.3.3.1.2 Pyrantel Tartrate for Prevention of Large Strongyles

Pyrantel tartrate is available as an alfalfa-based, pelleted formulation for inclusion in the daily ration. Continuous provision of pyrantel tartrate maintains drug concentrations within the gut lumen sufficient to kill ingested strongylid larvae before they are able to invade the gut wall and initiate migration.

Early dose titration studies determined that a daily dosage of 0.44 mg/kg did not achieve acceptable efficacy, but top-dress pellets providing 1.98−2.64 mg/kg were more than or equal to 98.3% effective in preventing establishment of *S. vulgaris* larvae. Subsequent dose confirmation studies demonstrated that two dosage forms, complete feed or top-dress pellets, were 99.7% and 98.3% effective, respectively, at preventing *S. vulgaris* larval infections [24].

In a controlled field study in Wisconsin, 56 mares and 39 foals were exposed to nematode infection by grazing infective pastures for approximately 1.5 years. Administration of daily pyrantel tartrate (2.64 mg/kg) was 100% effective in preventing *S. vulgaris* and *S. edentatus* infections compared to untreated controls [24]. In a more recent study, 28 young adult horses were inoculated with 25 infective *S. vulgaris* larvae weekly for 6 months. Administration of pyrantel tartrate (2.64 mg/kg) daily over the entire period reduced numbers of arterial larval stages by 98.7% in comparison to untreated controls [25].

4.3.3.1.3 Morantel Tartrate for Treatment of Large Strongyles

The label claims of most equine anthelmintics containing morantel tartrate are nearly identical to those in which the active agent is pyrantel pamoate/embonate, so routine indications and uses will not be discussed further. However, two combination products which contain morantel tartrate (Ammo Allwormer Paste; Moranox Broadspectrum Oral Worming Paste) have label claims against arterial stages of *S. vulgaris*. Undoubtedly, this larvicidal efficacy was achieved through the addition of abamectin or oxfendazole, respectively.

4.3.3.2 Small Strongyles (Cyathostominae)

As adults, all cyathostomins are found within the lumen of the equine large intestine. The route of infection for cyathostomins is the same as for large strongyles, but no systemic migration occurs within the host after ingested larvae invade the wall of the large intestine. Cyathostomin larvae develop within the mucosa or submucosa of the cecum, ventral colon and dorsal colon, where they are surrounded by a fibrous capsule of host origin. Ultimately, fourth-stage larvae emerge from the tissue cyst, enter the lumen of the gut, mature, and begin to reproduce. A typical prepatent period for small strongyles can vary from 6 weeks to more than 2 years.

Cyathostomin populations within an individual horse often number in the hundreds of thousands, yet these parasites are fairly innocuous and do not commonly cause severe clinical disease. However, if large numbers of encysted larvae emerge simultaneously, horses may develop a condition known as "larval cyathostominosis (LC)." This syndrome is characterized by generalized typhlocolitis, severe diarrhea, rapid weight loss, hypoproteinemia, and passage of large numbers of fourth-stage larvae in the feces. LC does not respond well to anthelmintic therapy and has a substantial mortality rate.

4.3.3.2.1 Pyrantel Pamoate/Embonate for Treatment of Cyathostomins

The common cyathostomins of managed horses or donkeys comprise at least 8 genera and 28 species [26], yet all are equally susceptible to pyrimidines in the absence of acquired resistance. In historical efficacy studies, pyrantel pamoate suspension at 6.6 mg/kg was 99% effective against pooled, mature cyathostomins, and approximately 90% effective against immature stages within the gut lumen (ie, L4s) [27]. It is important to note that pyrantel pamoate/embonate is not labeled for efficacy against luminal cyathostomin larvae (L4s), and this stage may survive pyrantel treatment while adults of the same species are fully susceptible.

LC is the most serious consequence of small strongyle infections in horses, and occurs when massive numbers of larvae emerge synchronously from the gut wall. Larval emergence may occur spontaneously due to seasonal or immunologic factors. However, the most common risk factor for LC is anthelmintic treatment within 2 weeks prior to the onset of clinical signs [28]. Removal of adult cyathostomins from the lumen apparently stimulates encysted larvae to resume maturation and emerge from their tissue cysts [29]. Most cases of LC involve horses less than 5 years of age that were treated with a nonlarvicidal anthelmintic during seasons when cyathostomin populations are in arrested development. Accordingly, practitioners should be cognizant of this potential complication when deworming young adult horses with pyrantel pamoate during seasons when local pasture transmission is minimal.

Some populations of cyathostomins have developed resistance to pyrimidines, as manifested by failures of the label dosage to reduce strongylid egg counts by more than 80% at 14 days posttreatment [30]. Pyrantel pamoate-resistant cyathostomin populations were first identified in Norway [31] and Louisiana [32]. A more recent coprologic survey conducted in the southeastern United States determined that cyathostomin populations were resistant to pyrantel pamoate in 40% of the horse herds tested [33].

4.3.3.2.2 Pyrantel Tartrate for Prevention of Cyathostomins
In a controlled field study in Wisconsin [24], daily administration of pyrantel tartrate for approximately 1.5 years reduced the numbers of all cyathostomin genera present by at least 99.7%. In a more recent study, 28 young adult horses were inoculated with 5000 infective larvae of a known, pyrantel-susceptible strain of cyathostomins on 5 days of each week for 6 months. Concurrent, daily administration of pyrantel tartrate (2.64 mg/kg) significantly reduced total counts of adult small strongyles by 93.0% ($P < 0.0001$) in comparison to untreated controls [25].

4.3.3.3 Ascarids (Parascaris spp.)
Horses acquire *Parascaris* infections by ingesting larvated eggs from the environment. Eggs hatch in the small intestine, and the liberated larvae penetrate the gut, migrate through the liver and lungs, and return to the small intestine approximately 1 month postinfection. Larvae continue their maturation within the lumen of the small intestine and eggs first appear in the feces about 75–90 days postinfection. Pulmonary symptoms may develop during systemic migration, but the presence of intestinal stages can result in poor growth, weight loss, and ill-thrift, especially

when worm burdens are large [34]. It was recently demonstrated that a majority of the equine ascarid isolates tested were *Parascaris univalens*, rather than *P. equorum* [35]. Distinctions between the two species are only feasible at the genetic level, so no differences in anthelmintic susceptibility are suspected.

4.3.3.3.1 Pyrantel Pamoate/Embonate for Treatment of Ascarids

Single doses of pyrantel pamoate (6.6—7.2 mg/kg in feed or via nasogastric tube) were 100% effective against immature *P. equorum*, and 92—100% effective against mature ascarids [22]. More recently, it was demonstrated that pyrantel pamoate paste (13.2 mg/kg) was 97.3% effective against adult *Parascaris* infections in foals which had been inoculated with a known, ML-resistant strain [36].

The most severe consequence of *Parascaris* infection is ascarid impaction, which is a mechanical blockage of the small intestinal lumen by large numbers of dead or living worms. Ascarid impactions most often occur within 48 h after effective deworming, especially when an anthelmintic with a neuromuscular mode of activity was used [37]. Practitioners should consider this potential adverse consequence when using pyrantel pamoate to treat sucklings and weanlings that might be harboring large ascarid burdens. An antemortem method for estimating the magnitude of ascarid burdens has been reported recently [38].

In 2008, Lyons et al. [39] reported that some *Parascaris* isolates in Kentucky were resistant to pyrantel pamoate in addition to MLs. Although Fecal Egg Count Reduction (FECR) Testing has only been validated for strongyles in horses, comparison of pre- and posttreatment ascarid egg counts should be useful for preliminary detection of resistant populations of *Parascaris*.

4.3.3.3.2 Pyrantel Tartrate for Prevention of Ascarids

In a controlled field study with naturally infected foals [24], daily treatment with 2.64 mg/kg pyrantel tartrate resulted in 100% reduction of adult and larval *P. equorum* numbers compared to controls.

4.3.3.4 Pinworms (Oxyuris equi)

Adult pinworms reside in the dorsal and descending colons, but gravid females migrate distally and deposit large egg masses in the perianal region. Eggs drop off into the environment and develop to the infective stage; new hosts are infected by ingestion of larvated eggs. The major clinical sign attributed to pinworm infection is anal pruritus and tail-rubbing associated with fecal egg deposition. Historically, pinworm infections caused problems only in juvenile horses, but that pattern has changed in recent years, perhaps due to genetic adaptations by *Oxyuris* populations [40].

4.3.3.4.1 Pyrantel Pamoate/Embonate for Treatment of Pinworms

A synopsis of historical efficacy studies of pyrantel pamoate against *Oxyuris equi* reported that most results ranged from 81% to 90% for both adult and larval stages [41]. Indeed, none of the anthelmintic classes tested to date in horses has consistently exhibited 100% activity against pinworms. A recent study with naturally infected horses demonstrated that pyrantel pamoate (13.2 mg/kg) was 91.2% and more than 99% effective against *O. equi* adults and fourth-stage larvae, respectively [42].

4.3.3.4.2 Pyrantel Tartrate for Prevention of Pinworms

In a controlled field study in Wisconsin with mares and foals exposed to natural infection [24], daily administration of pyrantel tartrate (2.64 mg/kg) for approximately 1.5 years reduced the numbers of pinworm fourth-stage larvae (L4s) by 97.8% and adults by 99.4%.

In attempting to manage putatively ML-resistant strains, some practitioners have achieved satisfactory control of *Oxyuris* infections by daily administration of pyrantel tartrate. However, this practice could eventually select for resistance to pyrimidine compounds [43].

4.3.3.5 Tapeworms (Anoplocephala perfoliata)

Anoplocephala perfoliata is the most prevalent tapeworm of managed horses. Adults reside in the cecum, in proximity to the ileocecal valve, and substantial inflammation develops within the gut wall at attachment sites. Most infections are asymptomatic, but tapeworm infection has been associated with ileocecal intussusceptions, ileal impactions, and a higher incidence of spasmodic colic [44].

4.3.3.5.1 Pyrantel Pamoate for Treatment of Tapeworms

Lyons et al. [45] reported that pyrantel pamoate (6.6 mg/kg) was 88% and 75% effective when administered as a paste or suspension formulation, respectively. The efficacy afforded by a dosage of 13.2 mg/kg was consistently more than or equal to 93% [46], and 19.8 mg/kg was reportedly 100% effective [47].

4.3.3.5.2 Pyrantel tartrate for Prevention of Tapeworms

In Florida, three horses with coprologically confirmed *Anoplocephala* infections received pyrantel tartrate (2.64 mg/kg) daily for 30 days. No tapeworms were found at necropsy, whereas an untreated pasture mate still harbored 12 specimens of *A. perfoliata* and one of *A. magna* [48]. In a subsequent herd study in Kentucky, 35 days of continuous, daily treatment with pyrantel tartrate reduced the proportion of fecal results that were positive for tapeworm eggs from 35% to 0% in 83 mares and from 33% to 2% in 58 yearlings [49]. Pyrantel tartrate has never earned a label claim for activity against equine cestodes.

4.3.4 General Considerations for Pyrimidines in Horses

Cyathostomins are the most prevalent internal parasites of mature horses, and are responsible for more than 98% of the strongyle eggs passed in the feces. Decisions to administer anthelmintic treatments to horses should be based on the results of quantitative fecal examination. In addition, comparing fecal egg counts before and after treatment is a simple method for monitoring the efficacy of such treatments. FECR can be calculated by comparing the pretreatment fecal egg count of an individual horse to the results of a sample collected 10−14 days posttreatment, thus:

$$\frac{EPG_{pre} - EPG_{post}}{EPG_{pre}} \times 100 = FECR, \text{ expressed as a percentage}$$

In horses, pyrantel pamoate is considered to be a "broad spectrum dewormer." This popular designation applies to equine anthelmintics which exhibit therapeutic efficacy against four distinct targets when administered at label dosages: large strongyles (subfamily Strongylinae), small strongyles (subfamily Cyathostominae), ascarids (*Parascaris* spp.), and pinworms (*Oxyuris equi*). Pyrantel pamoate has long been a staple of rotational deworming programs in which anthelmintics of different chemical classes and modes of activity are alternated between successive treatments. For nearly 50 years, one commonly employed strategy has been to repeat anthelmintic treatment of mature horses at 2-month intervals throughout the year (so-called "interval deworming"). This practice was based on a seminal report that strongyle egg counts remained low for approximately 8 weeks after treatment with thiabendazole [50]. It was recognized that by repeating treatment at predictable intervals, environmental contamination with worm eggs could be halted. Therefore, the strongylid life cycle would be disrupted, subsequent transmission diminished, and overall parasite burdens of participating horses subsequently reduced. This same program was eventually adopted for anthelmintics of different chemical classes, although the spectra and potential benefits of most alternative drugs differed substantially from those of the original therapeutic product, thiabendazole.

The 1966 rotational strategy was based on a parameter that has come to be known as the "egg reappearance period (ERP)." A modified definition for ERP is "the interval between treatment with an effective anthelmintic and resumption of egg counts of sufficient magnitude to decrease FECR below 80% for benzimidazole and pyrimidine anthelmintics, and below 90% for macrocyclic lactones" [30].

To determine the ERP for a pyrimidine drug in a specific horse population, FECR testing should be performed 2 weeks posttreatment and repeated at weekly intervals thereafter until the FECR falls below 80%. For example, if a horse had a pretreatment egg count of 1000 EPG, the ERP would expire on the earliest date when an egg count more than 200 EPG was recorded.

The current, expected ERP of pyrantel pamoate against susceptible strongyle populations is about 4 weeks [30], although 5—6 weeks was originally reported when the drug was first introduced [51,52]. Similar reductions of ERPs have been reported for all classes of equine anthelmintics that are currently marketed.

Herd and Gabel reported that egg reappearance periods were markedly shorter in juvenile horses, putatively due to temporal differences in parasite development and maturation as a consequence of incomplete acquired immunity [53].

Recently, simultaneous administration of pyrantel pamoate plus oxibendazole (ie, two anthelmintics of different chemical classes with overlapping nematocidal spectra) was shown to provide better FECR than either product used alone [54]. This combination approach provides another therapeutic alternative for equine parasite control in the face of increasing anthelmintic resistance. Similar combinations are already marketed in Australia, and include oral paste formulations containing pyrantel embonate plus ivermectin and praziquantel (Virbac Horse Wormer) or pyrantel embonate plus oxfendazole (Strategy-T).

4.3.5 Clinical Uses of Pyrimidines in Swine

Pyrantel tartrate
Morantel tartrate
Morantel citrate

4.3.5.1 Ascaris suum

The large roundworm of swine, *Ascaris suum*, is transmitted through ingestion of larvated eggs from the environment. Eggs hatch in the small intestine, larvae penetrate the gut wall and migrate progressively through the liver and lungs before returning to the gut. Larvae grow and mature in the small intestine, and eggs are passed in the feces approximately 6—8 weeks after infection. Although modern confinement management has greatly reduced transmission of ascarid infections, they have not been eliminated.

Adult ascarids in the gut usually do not cause dramatic clinical signs. Rather, their major impact is economic by contributing to poor feed conversion and diminished weight gains. Migrating *Ascaris* larvae may cause verminous pneumonia ("thumps") and scarring of the liver ("milk spots"). The latter circumstance often requires tissue condemnation at slaughter, with attendant economic losses.

4.3.5.1.1 Pyrantel Tartrate for Treatment and Prevention of Ascarids

Various regimens of pyrantel tartrate can be prepared and administered at different dosages to accomplish treatment and removal (1- or 3-day regimens) or prevention (continuous feeding) of ascarid infections. Therapeutic regimens are primarily used to alleviate clinical signs and to reduce environmental contamination with infective stages. Prophylactic regimens are employed to reduce systemic migration and its attendant productivity and economic impact.

4.3.5.1.2 Morantel Tartrate and Morantel Citrate for Treatment and Prevention of Ascarids

The label claims of porcine anthelmintics containing morantel citrate or morantel tartrate are similar to those in which the active agent is pyrantel tartrate, so routine indications and uses will not be discussed further. In Canada, Banminth II (morantel tartrate) has a unique label claim for efficacy against adults of the stomach worm *Hyostrongylus rubidus*.

4.3.5.2 *Oesophagostomum dentatum*

The nodular worm of swine, *O. dentatum*, is a large strongylate nematode that resides in the cecum and large intestine. Infection is transmitted through ingestion of infective, third-stage larvae. Larvae develop within the mucosa of the small and large intestines, and may undergo arrested development within nodules in the gut wall. Severe infections occasionally cause diarrhea, but the major effects are economic, as for *Ascaris*. The prepatent period may be as short as 3 weeks in swine managed intensively [55].

4.3.5.2.1 Pyrantel Tartrate for Treatment and Prevention of Nodular Worms

Most of the same regimens used for treatment or prevention of ascarids are also effective against nodular worms.

4.3.6 Clinical Uses of Pyrimidines in Sheep and Goats

Morantel tartrate
Morantel citrate

Nearly all of the major parasitic nematodes of sheep and goats are trichostrongylids; this family includes the genera *Haemonchus*, *Teladorsagia*, *Trichostrongylus*, *Nematodirus*, and *Cooperia*. This group consists of over one dozen species that differ in their preferred anatomic sites, pathogenicity, and economic importance. The only route of infection is ingestion of third-stage larvae, and prepatent periods are approximately 3 weeks. Several of the important trichostrongylids can undergo arrested development as an adaptation to unfavorable environmental or host conditions, and the anthelmintic susceptibility of arrested stages is generally much lower than that of adult stages. *Haemonchus contortus* is usually considered to be the single most important trichostrongylid of small ruminants because infections can be fatal, acquired immunity is incomplete, and anthelmintic resistance has rendered many drug classes ineffective.

4.3.6.1 *Morantel Tartrate and Morantel Citrate for Treatment of Small Ruminants*

Anthelmintic treatments of small ruminants are generally administered for one of three reasons: (1) to treat clinical disease; (2) to remove parasites or decrease transmission at specific, tactical times during the management cycle (eg, lambing or pre-weaning treatments); or (3) to reduce pasture contamination with trichostrongylid eggs and to maintain host health through repeated treatments at specific intervals during the grazing season.

The fact that pyrimidines cannot be administered by parenteral routes severely limits their use in all ruminants. The only options for delivery are individual, oral treatments, which are labor-intensive, or incorporation of medicinal products into feed. Rumatel 88 is the only pyrimidine approved as a feed additive for small ruminants [56], but it may not be available in some markets.

The apparent, unbounded genetic plasticity of *Haemonchus* enables many populations to develop acquired resistance to all classes of anthelmintics to which they are exposed with any frequency. Accordingly, anthelmintic failures and attendant clinical disease or production losses are the rule rather than the exception in small ruminants. Clinical haemonchosis can be especially problematic to manage because affected sheep or goats may be severely anemic, but individual treatment with a pyrimidine requires mustering and handling for oral administration. Such handling is inherently stressful, and mortality occasionally ensues among severely anemic animals that cannot meet the additional oxygen demands. The best and sometimes only option for treating clinical haemonchosis at the flock level is provision of an effective anthelmintic in the feed.

4.3.7 Clinical Uses of Pyrimidines in Cattle

Morantel Tartrate

As for other domestic ruminants, the major nematode parasites of cattle are trichostrongylids, and include the genera *Ostertagia*, *Trichostrongylus*, *Haemonchus*, *Nematodirus*, *Cooperia*, and *Dictyocaulus*. Of lesser importance are strongylids (*Oesophagostomum* spp.) and whipworms (*Trichuris* spp.). The trichostrongylids of cattle comprise nearly two dozen species that reside in the abomasum, small intestine, or lungs. Infection is acquired through ingestion of third-stage larvae, and prepatent periods are approximately 3 weeks. The major primary pathogens are *Ostertagia*, *Dictyocaulus*, and *Haemonchus*, although nearly all species have deleterious economic impact at some level. Other individual species can cause important clinical problems in isolated herds under unique management or environmental circumstances. All of the economically important trichostrongylids can undergo arrested development as an adaptation to host immunity or seasonal climatic conditions, and arrested stages are markedly less susceptible to most anthelmintics compared to mature worms.

To a greater extent than seen in small ruminants, mature cattle generally develop effective, albeit incomplete, acquired immunity to the major nematode pathogens. Another important distinction is that anthelmintic resistance among the trichostrongylids of cattle is a relatively recent development, and has been reported for *Cooperia* spp., *Haemonchus* spp., and *Ostertagia ostertagi* [57–60].

4.3.7.1 Morantel Tartrate for Treatment of Cattle

Historically, anthelmintic treatments were administered to individual cattle with evidence of clinical disease, or to entire herds when they were mustered for other management interventions, such as weaning or pregnancy evaluation [61]. Individual pyrimidine treatments (ie, Nematel boluses) would have been used under these circumstances, whereas feed additives (ie, Rumatel 88) were incorporated into the rations of some feedlot animals. Morantel tartrate was not always the best choice for some situations, however, because it has no efficacy against adult lungworms or against arrested stages of most nematodes, particularly *O. ostertagi*.

Traditional antiparasitic interventions were not based on sound epidemiologic principles, but the Paratect Cartridge and Paratect Flex Diffuser probably did more to advance the consideration of management conditions and seasonal transmission cycles in the practical control of bovine parasitism than any preceding commercial products. Indeed, the morantel sustained release devices spawned a revolution now known as the epidemiologic approach to parasite control in grazing animals. Both of these controlled release devices were designed to deliver continuous, therapeutic concentrations of morantel tartrate for at least 60 days after a single oral administration. This approach was shown to virtually halt nematode transmission in pasture venues, with previously unachievable enhancements of health and productivity [62,63]. In addition, valuable collateral information was gleaned regarding the pathogenicity of various individual nematode species, the development of host immunity to nematodes, and the economic potential of different management systems [64–66]. Interested readers are referred to the journal *Veterinary Parasitology*, 1983, Volume 12 (Issues 3, 4), which was a special issue dedicated to international, scientific evaluations of the morantel sustained release bolus.

Unfortunately, morantel tartrate never achieved its full commercial potential in cattle, largely because the avermectins were launched within the same decade. The appearance of ivermectin, with its high potency, unparalleled spectrum of efficacy, and ease of administration by oral, parenteral, or topical routes, virtually halted and even reversed any growth of the pyrimidine market for beef and dairy cattle. The subsequent approval of other ML anthelmintics for bovines (ie, abamectin, doramectin, eprino-mectin, moxidectin) and the current availability of generic ivermectin products have virtually halted the use of pyrimidines in cattle over the past 30 years. It remains to be seen whether the current interest in combination therapy (ie, two anthelmintics of different chemical classes with overlapping nematocidal spectra) will create a renewed demand for morantel tartrate, despite the requirement for labor-intensive, oral administration.

4.4 CONCLUSION

Anthelmintics of the pyrimidine class have been used widely for the past several decades to improve the health and productivity of every major species of domestic mammal. The universal success and acceptance of this drug class are due in no small part to the skills and innovations of untold numbers of chemists, pharmacologists, formulation scientists, and parasitologists around the world. Although anthelmintic resistance has emerged in some host–parasite systems, the pyrimidines will remain an essential fixture of the anthelmintic armamentarium for many years to come.

REFERENCES

[1] Roepstorff A, Bjorn H, Nansen P. Resistance of *Oesophagostomum* spp. in pigs to pyrantel citrate. Vet Parasitol 1987;24:229–39.
[2] Bjorn H, Hennessy DR, Friis C. The kinetic disposition of pyrantel citrate and pamoate and their efficacy against pyrantel-resistant *Oesophagostomum dentatum* in pigs. Int J Parasitol 1996;26:1375–80.
[3] Cardinal JR. Intraruminal controlled release boluses 2000 In: Rathbone MJ, Gurney R, editors. Controlled release veterinary drug delivery: biological and pharmaceutical considerations. Elsevier Science B.V.; 2000. p. 51–82
[4] Martin RJ, Clark CL, Trailovic SM, Robertson AP. Oxantel is an N-type (methyridine and nicotine) agonist not an L-type (levamisole and pyrantel) agonist: classification of cholinergic anthelmintics in *Ascaris*. Int J Parasitol 2004;34:1083–90.
[5] Reinemeyer CR, Faulkner CT, Assadi-Rad AM, Burr JH, Patton S. Comparison of the efficacies of three heartworm preventives against experimentally induced infections with *Ancylostoma caninum* and *Toxocara canis* in pups. J Am Vet Med Assoc 1995;206:1710–15.
[6] Little SE, Johnson EM, Lewis D, Jaklitsch RP, Payton ME, Blagburn BL, et al. Prevalence of intestinal parasites in pet dogs in the United States. Vet Parasitol 2009;166:144–52.
[7] Kalkofen UP. Hookworms of dogs and cats. In: Grieve RB, editor. Vet Clin N Am: Small Animal Practice. Philadelphia: W.B. Saunders Co; 1987. p. 1341–54.
[8] Efficacy of HeartGard® Plus. Freedom of information summary, HeartGard® Plus, <http://www.fda.gov/AnimalVeterinary/Products/ApprovedAnimalDrugProducts/FOIADrugSummaries/ucm054879.htm>; 2009 [accessed 27.09.15].

[9] Bowman DD, Montgomery SP, Zajac AM, Eberhard ML, Kazacos KR. Hookworms of dogs and cats as agents of cutaneous larva migrans. Trends Parasitol 2010;26:162—7.

[10] Parsons JC. Ascarid infections of cats and dogs. In: Grieve RB, editor. Vet Clin N Am: Small Animal Practice. Philadelphia: W.B. Saunders Co; 1987. p. 1307—39.

[11] Toxocara canis Control Recommendations. Companion Animal Parasite Council®, <http://www.capcvet.org/capc-recommendations/baylisascaris-procyonis-also-rac-coon-roundworm>; 2015 [accessed 27.09.15].

[12] Overgaauw PA, van Knapen F. Veterinary and public health aspects of *Toxocara* spp. Vet Parasitol 2013;193:398—403.

[13] Bauer C. Baylisascariosis-infections of animals and humans with 'unusual' round-worms. Vet Parasitol 2013;193:404—12.

[14] Baylisascaris procyonis Control Recommendations. Companion Animal Parasite Council®, <http://www.capcvet.org/capc-recommendations/baylisascaris-procyonis-also-raccoon-roundworm>; 2015 [accessed 27.09.15].

[15] Non-interference Studies of Drontal™ Plus. Freedom of Information Summary, Drontal™ Plus, <http://www.fda.gov/AnimalVeterinary/Products/ApprovedAnimal DrugProducts/FOIADrugSummaries/ucm054892.htm>; 2009 [accessed 27.09.15].

[16] Clark JA. *Physaloptera* stomach worms associated with chronic vomition in a dog in western Canada. Can Vet J 1990;31:12.

[17] Theisen SK, LeGrange SN, Johnson SE, Sherding RG, Willard MD. *Physaloptera* infection in 18 dogs with intermittent vomiting. J Am Anim Hosp Assoc 1988;34:74—8.

[18] Prevalence of Toxocara cati. Companion Animal Parasite Council®, <http://www. capcvet.org/capc-recommendations/ascarid-roundworm>; 2015 [accessed 27.09.15].

[19] Reinemeyer CR, DeNovo RC. Evaluation of the efficacy and safety of two formu-lations of pyrantel pamoate in cats. Am J Vet Res 1990;51:932—4.

[20] Prevalence of Feline Hookworms. Companion Animal Parasite Council®, <http://www.capcvet.org/capc-recommendations/hookworms>; 2015 [accessed 27.09.15].

[21] Santen DR, Chastain CB, Schmidt DA. Efficacy of pyrantel pamoate against *Physaloptera* in a cat. J Am Anim Hosp Assoc 1993;29:53—5.

[22] Lyons ET, Drudge JH, Tolliver SC. Critical tests of three salts of pyrantel against internal parasites of the horse. Am J Vet Res 1974;35:1515—22.

[23] Klei TR, Torbert BJ, Chapman MR, Ochoa R. Irradiated larval vaccinations of ponies against *Strongylus vulgaris*. J Parasitol 1982;68:561—9.

[24] Clinical Studies of Pyrantel Tartrate. Freedom of Information Summary, Strongid 48, <http://www.fda.gov/AnimalVeterinary/Products/ApprovedAnimalDrugProducts/ FOIADrugSummaries/ucm049922.htm>; 2009 [accessed 27.09.15].

[25] Reinemeyer CR, Prado JC, Nielsen MK, Schricker B, Kennedy T. Effects of daily pyrantel tartrate on strongylid population dynamics and performance parameters of young horses repeatedly infected with cyathostomins and *Strongylus vulgaris*. Vet Parasitol 2014;204:229—37.

[26] Tolliver SC. A practical method of identification of the North American Cyathostomes (Small Strongyles) in Kentucky. Kentucky Agricultural Experiment Station 2000;1—37 Bulletin SR-2000-1.

[27] Drudge JH, Tolliver SC, Lyons ET. Benzimidazole resistance of equine strongyles: critical tests of several classes of compounds against population B strongyles from 1977 to 1981. Am J Vet Res 1984;45:804—9.

[28] Reid SWJ, Mair TS, Hillyer MH, Love S. Epidemiological risk factors associated with a diagnosis of clinical cyathostomiasis in the horse. Eq Vet J 1995;27:127—30.

[29] Love S, Murphy D, Mellor D. Pathogenicity of cyathostome infection. Vet Parasitol 1999;85:113−22.

[30] Nielsen M.K., Mittel L., Grice A., Erskine M., Graves E., Vaala W., et al. AAEP parasite control guidelines. Am Assoc Eq Pract. <http://www.aaep.org/custdocs/ParasiteControlGuidelinesFinal.pdf>; 2013 [accessed 27.09.15].

[31] Ihler CF. A field survey on anthelmintic resistance in equine small strongyles in Norway. Acta Vet Scand 1995;36:135−43.

[32] Chapman MR, French DD, Monahan CM, Klei TR. Identification and characterization of a pyrantel pamoate-resistant cyathostome population. Vet Parasitol 1996;66:205−12.

[33] Kaplan RM, Klei TR, Lyons ET, Lester G, Courtney CH, French DD, et al. Prevalence of anthelmintic resistant cyathostomes on horse farms. J Am Vet Med Assoc 2004;225:903−10.

[34] Clayton HM. Ascarids: recent advances. In: Herd RP, editor. Vet Clin N Am: Equine Practice. Philadelphia: W.B. Saunders Co; 1986. p. 313−28.

[35] Nielsen MK, Wang J, Davis R, Bellaw JL, Lyons ET, Lear TL, et al. *Parascaris univalens*—a victim of large-scale misidentification? Parasitol Res 2014;113:4485−90.

[36] Reinemeyer CR, Prado JC, Nichols EC, Marchiondo AA. Efficacy of pyrantel pamoate against a macrocyclic lactone-resistant isolate of *Parascaris equorum* in horses. Vet Parasitol 2010;171:111−15.

[37] Cribb NC, Cote NM, Boure LP, Peregrine AS. Acute small intestinal obstruction associated with *Parascaris equorum* infection in young horses: 25 cases (1985−2004). N Z Vet J 2006;54:338−43.

[38] Nielsen MK, Donoghue EM, Stephens ML, Stowe CJ, Donecker JM, Fenger CK. An ultrasonographic scoring method for transabdominal monitoring of ascarid burdens in foals. Eq Vet J 2016;48:380−86.

[39] Lyons ET, Tolliver SC, Ionita M, Collins SS. Evaluation of parasiticidal activity of fenbendazole, ivermectin, oxibendazole, and pyrantel pamoate in horse foals with emphasis on ascarids (*Parascaris equorum*) in field studies on five farms in Central Kentucky in 2007. Parasitol Res 2008;103:287−91.

[40] Reinemeyer CR, Nielsen MK. Review of the biology and control of *Oxyuris equi*. Eq Vet Educ 2014;26:584−91.

[41] Reinemeyer CR. Anthelmintic resistance in non-strongylid parasites of horses. Vet Parasitol 2012;185:9−15.

[42] Reinemeyer CR, Prado JC, Nichols EC, Marchiondo AA. Efficacy of pyrantel pamoate and ivermectin paste formulations against naturally-acquired *Oxyuris equi* infections in horses. Vet Parasitol 2010;171:106−10.

[43] Brazik EL, Luquire JT, Little D. Pyrantel pamoate resistance in horses receiving daily administration of pyrantel tartrate 2006 J Am Vet Med Assoc 2006;228:101−3.

[44] Proudman CJ, French DD, Trees JA. Tapeworm infection is a significant risk factor for spasmodic colic and ileal impaction in the horse. Eq Vet J 1998;30:194−9.

[45] Lyons ET, Drudge JH, Tolliver SC. Pyrantel pamoate: evaluating its activity against equine tapeworms. Vet Med 1986;81:280−5.

[46] Reinemeyer CR, Hutchens DE, Eckblad WP, Marchiondo AA, Shugart JI. Dose-confirmation studies of the cestocidal activity of pyrantel pamoate paste in horses. Vet Parasitol 2006;138:234−9.

[47] Slocombe JOD. Prevalence and treatment of tapeworms in horses. Can Vet J 1979;20:136−40.

[48] Greiner EC, Lane TJ. Effects of the daily feeding of pyrantel tartrate on *Anoplocephala infections* in three horses: a pilot study. J Eq Vet Sci 1984;14:43−4.

[49] Lyons ET, Tolliver SC, McDowell KJ, Drudge JH. Field test of activity of the low dose rate (2.64 mg/kg) of pyrantel tartrate on *Anoplocephala perfoliata* in

Thoroughbreds on a farm in central Kentucky. J Helminthol Soc Wash 1997;64:283—5.

[50] Drudge JH, Lyons ET. Control of internal parasites of horses. J Am Vet Med Assoc 1966;148:378—83.

[51] Boersema JH, Borgsteede FHM, Eysker M, Saedt I. The reappearance of strongyle eggs in feces of horses treated with pyrantel embonate. Vet Quart 1995;17:18—20.

[52] Boersema JH, Eysker M, Maas J, van der Aar WM. Comparison of the reappearance of strongyle eggs in foals, yearlings, and adult horses after treatment with ivermectin or pyrantel. Vet Quart 1996;18:7—9.

[53] Herd RP, Gabel AA. Reduced efficacy of anthelmintics in young compared with adult horses. Eq Vet J 1990;22:164—9.

[54] Kaplan RM, West EM, Norat-Collazo LM, Vargas J. A combination treatment strategy using pyrantel pamoate and oxibendazole demonstrates additive effects for controlling equine cyathostomins. Eq Vet Educ 2014;26:485—91.

[55] Nansen P, Roepstorff A. Parasitic helminths of the pig: factors influencing transmission and infection levels. Int J Parasitol 1999;29:877—91.

[56] Reinemeyer CR, Pringle JK. Evaluation of the efficacy and safety of morantel tartrate in domestic goats. Vet Human Toxicol 1993;35:57—61 (supplement 2).

[57] Vermunt JJ, West DM, Pomroy WE. Multiple resistance to ivermectin and oxfendazole in *Cooperia* species of cattle in New Zealand. Vet Rec 1995;137:43—5.

[58] Gasbarre LC, Smith LL, Lichtenfels JR, Pilitt PA. The identification of cattle nematode parasites resistant to multiple classes of anthelmintics in a commercial cattle population in the US. Vet Parasitol 2009;166:281—5.

[59] Sutherland IA, Leathwick DM. Anthelmintic resistance in nematode parasites of cattle: a global issue? Trends Parasitol 2010;27:176—81.

[60] Edmonds MD, Johnson EG, Edmonds JD. Anthelmintic resistance of *Ostertagia ostertagi* and *Cooperia oncophora* to macrocyclic lactones in cattle from the western United States. Vet Parasitol 2010;174:224—9.

[61] McArthur MJ, Reinemeyer CR. Herding the U.S. cattle industry toward a paradigm shift in parasite control. Vet Parasitol 2014;204:34—43.

[62] Armour J, Bairden K, Duncan JL, Jones BM, Bliss DH. Studies on the control of bovine ostertagiasis using a morantel sustained-release bolus. Vet Rec 1981;108: 532—5.

[63] Brunsdon RV, Vlassoff A. A morantel sustained-release bolus for the control of gastro-intestinal nematodes in grazing calves. N Z Vet J 1981;29:139—41.

[64] Holmes PH, Bairden K, McKechnie D, Gettinby G, McWilliam PN. Effect of sustained release and pulse release anthelmintic intraruminal devices on development of pathophysiological changes and parasite populations in calves infected with *Ostertagia ostertagi* and *Cooperia oncophora*. Res Vet Sci 1991;51:223—6.

[65] Vercruysse J, Dorny P, Hilderson H, Berghen P. Efficacy of the morantel sustained-release trilaminate bolus against gastrointestinal nematodes and its influence on immunity in calves. Vet Parasitol 1992;44:97—106.

[66] Entrocasso CM, Parkins JJ, Armour J, Bairden K, McWilliam PN. Production, parasitological and carcase evaluation studies in steers exposed to trichostrongyle infection and treated with a morantel bolus or fenbendazole in two consecutive grazing seasons. Res Vet Sci 1986;40:76—85.

CHAPTER 5

Pyrantel Parasiticide Therapy in Humans

B. Levecke[1] and J. Vercruysse[2]
[1]Laboratory of Parasitology, Ghent University, Merelbeke, Belgium
[2]Ghent University Global Campus, Incheon Global Campus Foundation, Incheon, South Korea

5.1 INTRODUCTION

Today, the most important intestinal helminthiases are caused by *Ascaris lumbricoides* (roundworm), *Trichuris trichiura* (whipworm), *Ancylostoma duodenale* and *Necator americanus* (hookworms). These helminths are commonly known as soil-transmitted helminths (STHs), a name that refers to the role of the soil in the transmission of these helminth species. Infected individuals will contaminate the soil with feces containing helminth eggs. In the soil an infectious larval stage will develop in the eggs. Infection of individuals is by ingestion of eggs containing larvae through food or dirty hands, or by larvae penetrating the skin (hookworms). Finally, larvae develop into adult worms in the intestine, which produce eggs that are passed in stool [1].

Soil-transmitted helminthiasis occurs throughout the developing world and remains a major public health problem in the poorest communities with enormous consequences on health and development of preschool and school age children. It is estimated that STHs affect approximately 1.4 billion people worldwide, and the greatest numbers of infections occur in sub-Saharan Africa, the Americas, China, and East Asia [2]. The morbidity caused by these worms is commonly associated with heavy infection intensities. Preschool age and school age children are the most vulnerable group and they harbor the greatest numbers of intestinal worms. As a result, they experience growth stunting and diminished physical fitness as well as impaired memory and cognition [1,3,4]. These adverse health consequences combine to impair childhood educational performance and reduce school attendance [5,6]. To fight these helminthiases, the World Health Assembly passed a resolution in 2001 (WHA54.19) urging member states to control the morbidity of STH infections through large-scale use of anthelmintic drugs in countries where STHs are endemic.

In the present chapter, we first briefly discuss the current global strategy to control soil-transmitted helminthiasis. Next, we review the therapeutic efficacy of pyrantel (PYR) reported in literature against these helminthiases, both as a mono and a combination therapy followed by the current status of anthelmintic resistance in human STHs. Finally, we discuss the role of PYR as a large-scale administration drug to control soil-transmitted helminthiasis.

5.2 CURRENT GLOBAL STRATEGY TO CONTROL HUMAN SOIL-TRANSMITTED HELMINTHIASIS

The global strategy for the control of soil-transmitted helminthiasis is preventive chemotherapy (PC) whereby anthelminthic drugs are periodically administered to at-risk populations, usually without prior diagnosis [7−9]. For the control of soil-transmitted helminthiasis, World Health Organization (WHO) recommends a school-based control strategy that mainly targets school age children, but that also encourages targeting other high-risk groups, such as preschool age children and pregnant women. The frequency of these programs depends on the initial prevalence, drugs being administered annually when the prevalence is at least 20%, and biannually when the prevalence exceeds 50%. When the prevalence is below 20% it is not recommended to implement PC, instead a case-to-case treatment should be applied [9]. To date, the four WHO essential anthelminthic drugs against soil-transmitted helminthiasis are albendazole (ALB; 400 mg), levamisole (LEV; 80 mg or 2.5 mg/kg), mebendazole (MEB; 500 mg), and PYR (10 mg/kg) [9].

However, the two drugs commonly used nowadays are ALB and MEB. These drugs belong to the same pharmacological family (benzimidazole (BZ) drugs), and are currently made available to WHO through donations of pharmaceutical industry. Both drugs are highly efficacious against *A. lumbricoides* (>97%), ALB is more efficacious against hookworm (96% vs 80%), and both drugs are unsatisfactory when used as a single regimen against *T. trichiura* infection (~63%) [10,11]. Moreover, therapeutic efficacy can vary across levels of infection intensity, ALB showing a high efficacy when the intensity of *T. trichiura* is low and poor efficacy when infection levels are high [12]. Despite these differences in efficacy between both drugs and STH species, it is important to note that practical experience with both drugs in the field over several years indicates that both are equally effective in controlling all three STH species irrespective of their initial prevalence and intensity of infection [13–15].

Recently, this control strategy has received increased political and scientific attention. The WHO has devised a roadmap to guide implementation of the policies and strategies set out in a global plan to combat Neglected Tropical Diseases (NTDs) (period 2008–15) [16], and more than 70 pharmaceutical companies, governments, and global health organizations committed to supporting this roadmap in the London Declaration on NTDs in January 2012 by sustaining or expanding drug donation programs [17]. For example, the number of ALB and MEB tablets donated for control of soil-transmitted helminthiasis only increased from approximately 210 million tablets in 2012 to 370 million in 2015 [18]. With this growing attention, WHO aims to increase the coverage of the preschool and school aged children in need of drug administration from approximately 34% (estimated coverage in 2013 [18]) to at least 75% by 2020, and to ultimately eliminate soil-transmitted helminthiasis as a public health problem in children [19]. However, these worldwide prospects for increased coverage warrant caution. PC programs to control soil-transmitted helminthiasis predominantly rely on just one group of drugs, the BZ drugs, which, as substantiated in veterinary medicine, make these campaigns highly vulnerable to the development of anthelminthic resistance (AR) [20–22]. As a consequence of this, it will be essential that efficacy of drugs are periodically assessed to detect emerging AR.

Drug efficacy can be summarized either qualitatively or quantitatively. Qualitative metrics are based on the absence or presence of helminth eggs in stool, and result in cure rate (CR) estimates, whereas quantitative metrics are based on the enumeration of helminth eggs in stool, and include egg reduction rate (ERR) estimates. However, there is ongoing debate whether CR is an appropriate metric to assess drug efficacy as opposed to ERR [23,24]. Vercruysse and collaborators also highlighted that the probability of finding zero eggs after drug administration increases as a function of decreasing infection intensity at baseline [10]. As a result, comparisons between populations differing in infection intensity at baseline are biased to provide different conclusions about drug efficacy when summarized by means of CR. More recently it has been shown that CR is affected by both sampling (collection of stools over consecutive days) and diagnostic effort (multiple readings per stool sample), but that this was not the case for estimating ERR [25].

To encourage monitoring of efficacy drugs administered in PC programs in a standardized manner, the WHO has recently published guidelines on how to assess drug efficacy against helminthiasis, such as STH [26]. This document provides up-to-date guidance on (1) when to assess the efficacy of drugs; (2) how a drug efficacy should be assessed, including detailed recommendations on indicator of drug efficacy, sample size, follow-up period, laboratory methods, statistical analysis, and final interpretation of the observed drug efficacy; and (3) how to respond when drug efficacy is unsatisfactory.

5.3 THERAPEUTIC EFFICACY OF PYR AGAINST HUMAN SOIL-TRANSMITTED HELMINTHIASIS

The scientific interest for PYR in human anthelminthic therapy originates from the promising efficacy results against experimental hookworm (*Ancylostoma caninum*) infections in dogs reported by Cornwell and Jones in 1968 [27]. In the years that have followed, various regimens of the drug have been validated against a variety of human intestinal helminthiasis, including but not limited to the human hookworms [28–30]. Among other intestinal helminthiasis for which the activity of PYR was evaluated in the early 1970s were pinworms (*Enterobious vermicularis*) [31,32], roundworms [28,33], whipworms [28,34], wireworms (*Trichostrongylus*) [35,36], and threadworms (*Strongyloides*) [28,36]. Following these early trials, the efficacy of PYR was further explored in combination with MEB [37–39] and oxantel (OX) [40,41], at that time novel anthelminthic drugs. The main rationale of these combination therapies was to prevent erratic ascariasis following MEB treatment, as PYR paralyzes worms [42], and to increase the activity against whipworm infections, as OX is more potent to kill whipworms (see section: Combination Therapy).

PYR was added to WHO's Essential Medicines List (EML) in 1983, and together with MEB, niclosamide, and praziquantel, which were added to the initial WHO EML of 1977, it is one of the first essential medicines for intestinal helminthiasis that remains listed in the current EML. Other current essential medicines for intestinal helminthiasis listed are ALB and LEV [43].

The therapeutic efficacy of PYR has been previously reviewed by Janssens [42], and by Keiser and Utzinger [44]. Besides the obvious difference in time frame in which they reviewed trials (Janssens [42]: from 1969 to 1981; Keiser and Utzinger [44]: from 1960 to 2007), these two reviews were assessed with different goals. Janssens [42] aimed to summarize efficacy PYR against a wide range of helminthiasis regardless of the dosage and study design (randomized controlled vs observational trials), whereas Keiser and Utzinger [44] focused on randomized controlled trials evaluating the efficacy of a single-oral dose PYR 10 mg/kg against soil-transmitted helminthiasis only. In this chapter we will summarize the efficacy of all dosages of PYR evaluated against the four STH species, either as a mono or a combination therapy, between the period 1966–2015.

We searched PubMed (http://www.ncbi.nlm.nih.gov) (1966 to February 2015), ISI Web of Science (http://www.isiknowledge.com) (1960 to February 2015) and ScienceDirect (http://www.sciencedirect.com) (1960 to February 2015). No restrictions were set on year of publication, but publications published in any other language than English, French, Spanish, or Portuguese were not considered. We used the terms *pyrantel pamoate* in combination with ascariasis, *A. lumbricoides*, hookworm, *An. duodenale*, *N. americanus*, trichuriasis, *T. trichiura*, and *soil-transmitted helminths*. We were interested in CR and ERR as a measure of drug efficacy.

It is important to note that the efficacy data available have been obtained through a variety of widely differing study protocols, including protocols that used different diagnostic methods (eg, formol-ether concentration, Kato-Katz thick smear, McMaster, Stoll's method, Willis flotation technique), stool collection strategy (single stool sample vs 24 h stool for consecutive days), different durations in follow-up periods (7–61 days), different study populations (children vs adults) with varying level of infection intensity (25th (Q25) and 75th (Q75) quantile of mean fecal egg counts at baseline: *A. lumbricoides*: 6413–36,808 eggs per gram of stool (EPG); *T. trichiura*: 912–6,330 EPG; hookworm: 873–4,341 EPG) and statistical analyses (different formula to calculate ERR [45]). Hence, a ready comparison of the different trials is difficult to impossible, and consequently impedes a robust analysis of drug efficacy (see also Keiser and Utzinger [44]). In addition, the drug efficacy is mostly reported as CR, but recent studies highlight that this is not the recommended metric to summarize drug efficacy, and that the ERR should be applied instead [10,23,25,26].

5.3.1 Mono Therapy

We found 199 trials in which PYR was evaluated as a mono therapy. Overall, PYR was evaluated across different dosages and/or days of administration. In the majority of the trials dosage of PYR was based on body weight, dosages ranging from 2.2 [28,46] to 100 mg/kg [47]. In the minority of the trials ($n = 8$), a fixed dose was administered (500 mg) [39], 100 mg twice a day for 3 days [48], 750 mg [49,50], and 1100 mg [51]. We will focus only on trials in which PYR was dosed based on body weight. Table 5.1 summarizes the different PYR regimens that have been evaluated for the different STH species, resulting in 87 trials for hookworms, 67 for *A. lumbricoides*, and 37 for *T. trichiura*.

Various studies have assessed the dose-response for a single-oral dose PYR for the different STH species either for 1 day [30,33,36,46,52−55] or for consecutive days [30,32,54,56−59]. Fig. 5.1 illustrates the dose−response for a single-oral dose PYR administered for 1 day, indicating that the efficacy varied considerably across the different dosages. This was in particular for *A. lumbricoides*, for which the efficacy linearly increased between a dose of 2.5 mg/kg and 10 mg/kg, but remained unchanged when the dose exceeded 10 mg/kg. Although less pronounced, a similar trend was observed for hookworms, justifying the recommended dose of 10 mg/kg. For *T. trichiura*, no clear conclusions could be drawn, as only two studies assessed the dose−response for this

Table 5.1 The number of trials evaluating a mono therapy of PYR for *A. lumbricoides*, *T. trichiura*, and hookworms

Dosage	*A. lumbricoides*	*T. trichiura*	Hookworms
2.2−8.7 mg/kg	14	4	11
1 day	3	12	9
2−3 days	1	2	2
10.0−11.0 mg/kg	42	22	38
1 day	14	35	25
2−3 days	8	7	13
14.0−17.4 mg/kg	2	0	8
1 day	0	2	8
2−3 days	0	0	0
20.0−22.0 mg/kg	7	9	21
1 day	2	2	10
2−3 days	7	5	11
≥33.0 mg/kg	2	2	9
1 day	1	1	7
2−3 days	1	1	2
Total	67	37	87

When the dosage ranged between two numbers (eg, 8.5−10 mg/kg), the trial was classified in the highest dosage (*in casu* 10 mg/kg).

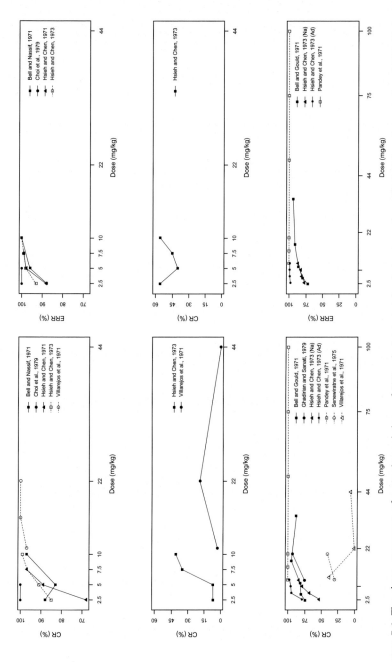

Figure 5.1 The dose–response of a single oral dose of PYR administered for 1 day based on CR (left hand graphs) and ERR (right hand graphs) for *A. lumbricoides* (top graphs), *T. trichiura* (middle graphs), and hookworms (bottom graphs).

parasite. The dose—response of PYR administered over consecutive days for PYR approximately 10 mg/kg is summarized in Fig. 5.2, the dose—response for approximately 20 mg/kg is summarized in Fig. 5.3. Overall, there is an increase in efficacy as a function of number of days of drug administration. However, this increase in efficacy varies between trials (lines representing trials across each other), STH species (lines representing ERR are steep for *T. trichiura*, and flat for *A. lumbricoides*), and metrics of efficacy (CR vs ERR).

Fig. 5.4 illustrates the efficacy measured as CR ($n = 71$) and ERR ($n = 34$) for a single oral dose approximately 10 mg/kg PYR, the WHO recommended dosage for STH, indicating that PYR is highly efficacious against roundworms ($n = 34$, median CR = 96.0% [Q25; Q75: 90.3; 99.0]; $n = 16$, median ERR = 98.5% [Q25; Q75: 94.8; 99.3]), shows moderate efficacy against hookworms (median CR = 54.5% [Q25; Q75: 34.5; 81.8], $n = 24$: median ERR = 67.0% [Q25; Q75: 62.5; 89.5], $n = 11$), and has poor efficacy against whipworm infections (median CR = 19.0% [Q25; Q75: 4; 41], $n = 13$; median ERR = 48.0% [Q25; Q75: 14; 64.0], $n = 7$).

5.3.2 Combination Therapy

PYR has been evaluated in combination with MEB and OX, the latter combination receiving the most attention for its activity against whipworms. We found 68 trials in which PYR was evaluated in combination with OX. As for PYR administered as a mono therapy, different dosages of PYR/OX were evaluated against STH species, ranging from a single oral dose of 50 mg [42] to 15—20 mg/kg for three consecutive days (eg, 40). Table 5.2 summarizes the different PYR/OX regimens based on body weight that have been evaluated for the different STH species, resulting in 23 trials for *T. trichiura*, 21 for hookworms, and 20 for *A. lumbricoides*.

A head-to-head comparison of PYR and PYR/OX, administered as a 10 mg/kg dose, is reported by Sinniah and Sinniah [59]. The results for *T. trichiura* and hookworm are graphically illustrated in Fig. 5.5. For *T. trichiura* a single oral dose of PYR/OX (CR = 48%; ERR = 86%) was almost as efficacious as a single oral dose of PYR administered for three consecutive days (CR = 58%; ERR = 89%). For hookworms the added value was small, the combination resulting in slightly (ERR) to

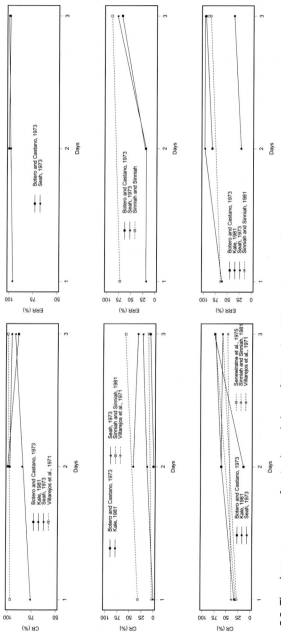

Figure 5.2 The dose–response of a single oral dose of 10 mg/kg PYR administered for consecutive days based on CR (left hand graphs) and ERR (right hand graphs) for *A. lumbricoides* (top graphs), *T. trichiura* (middle graphs), and hookworms (bottom graphs).

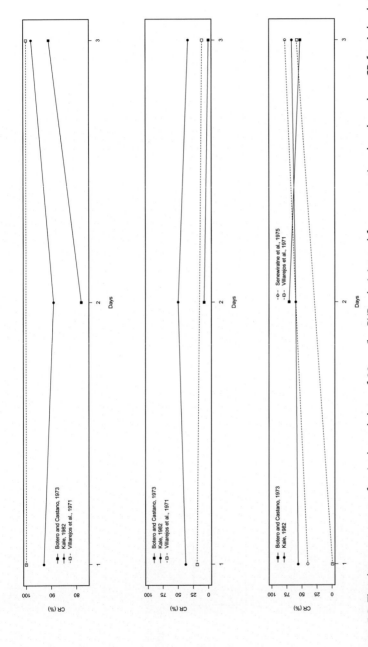

Figure 5.3 The dose—response of a single oral dose of 20 mg/kg PYR administered for consecutive days based on CR for *A. lumbricoides* (top graph), *T. trichiura* (middle graph), and hookworms (bottom graph).

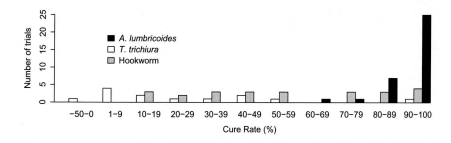

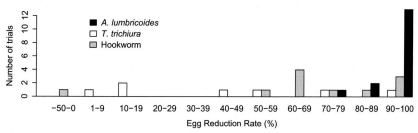

Figure 5.4 The efficacy of a single oral dose of 10 mg/kg PYR administered for 1 day measured as CR (top graph) and ERR (bottom graph) against *A. lumbricoides*, *T. trichiura*, and hookworm.

moderately higher (CR) efficacy results compared to a mono therapy. The difference in CR between PYR and PYR/OX was 8% when drugs were administered for 1 day, but 24% when drugs were administered for three consecutive days. The difference in ERR between drugs was approximately 5%. For *A. lumbricoides*, the added value is negligible, as both drugs were highly efficacious when administered for 1 day (PYR: CR = 96%, ERR = 98% vs PYR/OX: CR = 98%, ERR = 99%).

Overall 10 mg/kg of PYR/OX is highly efficacious against roundworms (median CR = 97.0% [Q25; Q75: 96.3; 97.0], n = 6) and shows moderate efficacy against both hookworms (median CR = 73.0% [Q25; Q75: 45.0; 89.0], n = 9) and whipworm infections (median CR = 60.5% [Q25; Q75: 40.5; 74.5], n = 6). These results confirm that combining PYR/OX widens the spectrum of PYR mainly against whipworms, and to a lesser extent against hookworms.

Combination therapy PYR and MEB has been evaluated against STH in seven trials (*A. lumbricoides* [37–39]; *T. trichiura* and hookworms [37,38]).

Table 5.2 The number of trials evaluating PYR in combination with OX for
A. lumbricoides, *T. trichiura*, and hookworms

Dosage	A. lumbricoides	T. trichiura	Hookworms
10 mg/kg	6	7	9
1 day	6	6	8
2–3 days	1	0	1
15 mg/kg	4	5	3
1 day	3	2	2
2–3 days	2	2	1
20 mg/kg	9	11	9
1 day	6	4	4
2–3 days	5	5	5
30 mg/kg	1	0	0
1 day	0	1	0
2–3 days	0	0	0
Total	20	23	21

When the dosage ranged between two numbers (eg, 15–20 mg/kg), the trial was classified in the highest dosage (*in casu* 20 mg/kg).

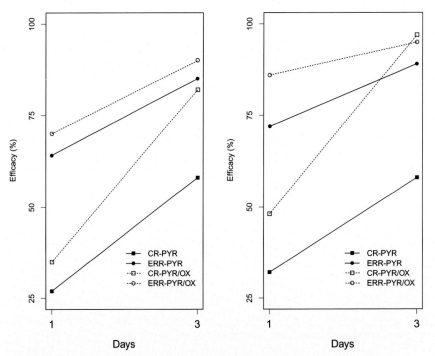

Figure 5.5 The efficacy measured as CR and ERR of PYR in a mono therapy and in combination with OX administered at a dose of 10 mg/kg for one and three consecutive days against hookworm (left hand graph) and *T. trichiura* (right hand graph). These data were reported by Sinniah and Sinniah [59].

The combination was administered in different dosages of 60 mg/kg PYR and 200 mg MEB for 3 days [37]; 150 mg PYR and 100 mg MEB b.i.d. for 3 days [38]; 200 mg PYR in co-administration with 200 mg MEB [39]. With the exception of a CR of 69% against *T. trichiura* (150 mg PYR and 100 mg MEB twice a day for 3 days [39], each of these regiments resulted in high CRs (≥98%). In one trial PYR (10 mg/kg), OX (10 mg/kg), and MEB (100 mg) were administered as one combination [60], resulting in high efficacy against *A. lumbricoides* (CR = ERR = 100%) and *T. trichiura* (CR = 81%, ERR = 94%), and moderate high efficacy against hookworm (CR = 67%, ERR = 86%).

5.4 ROLE OF PYR AS A MASS ADMINISTRATION DRUG

From the 1970s onward PYR has been extensively used in numerous STH control programs, particularly in Asian countries. Examples of countries that periodically administered PYR in the early phase of their national PC program are Indonesia, the Republic of Korea, and the Philippines [61]. In the majority of the programs PYR was administered as a mono therapy (10 mg/kg), a combination therapy with OX was also applied in Indonesia to increase the impact on *T. trichiura* infections [61]. However, over time the BZ drugs gradually replaced PYR as the drug of choice in MDA programs to control STHs. For example, in the Republic of Korea, where STH has been successfully eliminated as a public health problem, PYR was administered for 15 years (1973−88) of the 25 years of PC (1969−95), but was replaced by BZ drugs in the final years of the campaign (MEB: 1983−93; ALB: 1988−95) [62]. This worldwide shift from PYR to BZ can been explained by a variety of factors, but the most important is probably the administration of BZ without the need for weighing of the subjects.

This dominance of BZ in PC programs, however, does not imply that the role of PYR as a MDA drug is nonexisting. On the contrary, we now rely on two drugs of the same class and with the same mode of action (the inhibition of the polymerization of microtubules), and hence the emergence of AR as drug donations expand is likely to occur. Moreover, development of AR against one BZ drug would most likely be accompanied by poor anthelmintic drug efficacy of the other BZ drug. As a matter of fact there is a paucity of anthelmintic drugs that are both licensed for the treatment of STH infections in humans and that are commercially available [63,64], and hence should AR against BZ drugs eventually emerge and spread, MDA-based control of STH will be even more limited than at present with few acceptable alternative options.

A potential back-up drug is PYR in combination with PYR/OX, this is for three reasons. First, this drug combination has a mode of action different to BZ drugs, and hence allows controlling STHs where BZs are failing. Second, combining the drugs allows a broadening of the spectrum of STHs (see section: Combination Therapy). Third, a drug combination would not only broaden the spectrum, but more importantly it will also delay the development of AR. It has been shown both in simulation and in empirical studies that combining drugs will delay AR in animal STH [65–68]. For example, a field study indicated that the clinical efficacy of ivermective (IVM) against STH in sheep, which were experimental infected with both susceptible (IVM and LEV) and resistant strains (IVM), dropped from approximately 93% to approximately 75% in a period of 2 years when sheep where monthly dosed with IVM alone, but from approximately 99% to approximately 93% when IVM was combined with LEV [69]. In addition to this field study, a simulation study was conducted to assess the impact of initial frequency of AR. The results of this simulation study indicated that the impact of combination drugs on the development of AR against IVM depends on the initial frequency of AR genes. When the initial frequency was low ($=0.026$) the gene frequency after approximately 2.5 years was 0.14 times smaller in the animals receiving IVM/LEV compared to animals that received IVM alone. However, when the initial frequency was high ($=0.175$), the gene frequency after approximately 2.5 years was only 0.65 times smaller.

5.5 ANTHELMINTIC RESISTANCE

The possible development of AR to currently available anthelmintics is a subject of considerable interest from both an animal and public health point of view. The fear of AR developing in human STH is based on the experience of veterinary medicine. In livestock, resistance to the five major anthelmintic families, including BZ, imidazothiazoles/tetrahydroxypyrimidines, macrocyclic lactones, amino-acetonitrile derivates, and spiroindoles, is widespread, and has been extensively studied. PYR resistance has been described for *An. caninum* in Australian dogs [70], *Oesophagostomum dentatum* in intensively farmed pig herds in Denmark [71], and numerous reports indicating the emergence of PYR resistance in intestinal helminths of horses [72–74]. In humans only one study reported potential AR in hookworms (*Ancylostoma*) against PYR in closed Aborginal communities (Australia) [75]. In these communities, the efficacy of PYR dropped from almost 100% to less than 50% (CR: 15%; ERR: 45%) over a period of approximately a decade. Because of the high efficacy of ALB (100%), which had not been used before, the most likely reason for the failure of PYR in the treatment of *Ancylostoma* was the development of resistance as a consequence of the frequent administration of the drug. However, the low number of patients ($n = 15$) and the high pretreatment egg counts (mean baseline FEC $= 869$ EPG) may have affected the estimate of efficacy, and hence the final conclusions drawn.

Currently there are thus no conclusive data that AR against PYR (and other anthelmintics) is widespread for STH. However, we should also consider the lack of tools and investigations, demonstrating that putative resistance alleles have increased in frequency in human STH following anthelmintic treatment, and none that these alleles have spread in the parasite populations. Moreover it will be very important that future studies monitoring AR differentiate a reduced efficacy from AR, though in practice it is not at all easy to do so. Many potential factors may affect the efficacy of an anthelmintic, and should first be excluded before AR can be assumed. Such issues have been extensively investigated in veterinary intestinal nematode infections, but less so among species infecting humans [10].

Finally, it will be important to further preserve the efficacy of anthelmintic drugs and to delay the emergence of AR. Combining of drugs with different modes of action is therefore recommended. Combining anthelmintic drugs is widespread in veterinary medicine and now also receives due attention for human STHs as illustrated by the increased number of studies evaluating drug combinations, particularly against human *T. trichiura* infections. For example, drugs that have been combined with BZ are LEV [76], IVM [77–82], nitazoxanide [83], and OX [82,84].

5.6 CONCLUSIONS

Today, STHs occur throughout the developing world and remain a major public health problem in the poorest communities with enormous consequences on the health and development of children. Although PYR has been outcompeted as a drug of choice to control these infections, it may play a crucial role, preferable in combination with OX, in the upcoming era of intensified drug donations. Current control programs only rely on a few drugs, and there is a paucity of drugs that are both licensed for the treatment of STH infections in humans and that are commercially available. However, large-scale trials are needed to evaluate the efficacy of PYR/OX against STHs measured as ERR in a wide range of endemic countries and to persuade the pharmaceutical industry to continue production.

REFERENCES

[1] Bethony JM, Brooker SJ, Albonico M, Geiger SM, Loukas A, Diemert D, et al. Soil-transmitted helminth infections: ascariasis, trichuriasis, and hookworm. Lancet 2006;367:1521−32.
[2] Pullan RL, Smith JL, Jasrasaria R, Brooker SJ. Global numbers of infection and disease burden of soil-transmitted helminth infections in 2010. Parasit Vectors 2014;7:37.
[3] Crompton DWT, Nesheim MC. Nutritional impact of intestinal helminthiasis during the human life cycle. Ann Rev Nutr 2002;22:35−59.
[4] Stephenson LS, Latham MC, Ottesen EA. Malnutrition and parasitic helminth infections. Parasitology 2000;121:S23−8.
[5] Miguel E, Kremer M. Worms: identifying impacts on education and health in the presence of treatment externalities. Econometrica 2004;72:159−217.
[6] Hotez PJ, Brindley PJ, Bethony JM, King CH, Pearce EJ, Jacobson J. Helminth infections: the great neglected tropical diseases. J Clin Invest 2008;118:1311−21.
[7] World Health Organization. Preventive chemotherapy in human helminthiasis: coordinated use of anthelminthic drugs in control interventions: a manual for health professionals and programme managers. Geneva, Switzerland: World Health Organization; 2006.
[8] World Health Organization. First WHO report on neglected tropical diseases 2010: working to overcome the global impact of neglected tropical diseases. Geneva, Switzerland: World Health Organization; 2010.
[9] World Health Organization. Helminth control in school-age children: a guide for managers of control programmes. 2nd ed. Geneva, Switzerland: World Health Organization; 2011.
[10] Vercruysse J, Behnke JM, Albonico M, ShaaliMakame A, Angebault C, Bethony JM, et al. Assessment of the anthelmintic efficacy of albendazole in school children in seven countries where soil-transmitted helminths are endemic. PLoS Negl Trop Dis 2011;5:e948.
[11] Levecke B, Montresor A, Albonico M, Ame SM, Behnke JM, Bethony JM, et al. Assessment of anthelmintic efficacy of mebendazole in school children in six countries where soil-transmitted helminthsare endemic. PLoS Negl Trop Dis 2014;8: e3204.
[12] Levecke B, Mekonnen Z, Albonico Z, Vercruysse J. The impact of baseline FEC on the efficacy of a single-dose albendazole against *Trichuris trichiura*. Trans R Soc Trop Med Hyg 2012;106:128−30.
[13] Sinuon M, Tsuyuoka R, Socheat D, Odermatt P, Ohmae H, Matsuda H, et al. Control of *Schistosoma mekongi* in Cambodia: results of eight years of control activities in the two endemic provinces. Trans R Soc Trop Med Hyg 2006;101:34−9.

[14] Flisser A, Valdespino JL, Garcia-Garcia L, Guzmán-Bracho C, Aguirre Alcántara MT, Mañon ML, et al. Using national health weeks to deliver deworming to children: lessons from Mexico. J Epidemiol Community Health 2008;62:314−17.

[15] Tun A, Myat SM, Gabrielli AF, Montresor A. Control of soil transmitted helminthiasis in Myanmar. Result of 7 years of deworming. Trop Med Int Health 2013;18:1017−20.

[16] World Health Organization. Accelerating work to overcome the global impact of neglected tropical diseases: a roadmap for implementation. Geneva, Switzerland: World Health Organization; 2012.

[17] NTD Partner Website. Uniting to combat neglected tropical diseases. Ending the neglect and reaching 2020 goals, <http://www.unitingtocombatntds.org>; 2014 [accessed 01.02.14].

[18] World Health Organization. Soil-transmitted helminthiases: number of children treated in 2013. Week Epidemiol Rec 2015;90:89−96.

[19] World Health Organization. Soil-transmitted helminthiases: eliminating soil-transmitted helminthiases as a public health problem in children: progress report 2001−2010 and strategic plan 2011−2020. Geneva, Switzerland: World Health Organization; 2012.

[20] Geerts S, Gryseels B. Drug resistance in human helminths: current situation and lessons from livestock. Clin Microbiol Rev 2000;13:202−22.

[21] Albonico M, Engels D, Savioli L. Monitoring drug efficacy and early detection of drug resistance in human soil-transmitted nematodes: a pressing public health agenda for helminth control. Int J Parasitol 2004;34:1205−10.

[22] Vercruysse J, Albonico M, Behnke JM, Kotze AC, Prichard RK, McCarthy JS, et al. Is anthelmintic resistance a concern for the control of human soil-transmitted helminths? Int J Parasitol Drugs Drug Resist 2011;1:14−27.

[23] Montresor A. Cure rate is not a valid indicator for assessing drug efficacy and impact of preventive chemotherapy interventions against schistosomiasis and soil-transmitted helminthiasis. Trans R Soc Trop Med Hyg 2011;105:361−3.

[24] Montresor A, Engels D, Chitsulo L, Gabrielli A, Albonico M, Savioli L, et al. The appropriate indicator should be used to assess treatment failure in STH infections. Am J Trop Med Hyg 2011;85:579−80.

[25] Levecke B, Brooker SJ, Knopp S, Steinmann P, Stothard RJ, Sousa-Figueiredo JC, et al. Effect of sampling and diagnostic effort on the assessment of schistosomiasis and soil-transmitted helminthiasis and drug efficacy: a meta-analysis of six drug efficacy trials and one epidemiological survey. Parasitology 2014;141:826−40.

[26] World Health Organization. Assessing the efficacy of anthelminthic drugs against schistosomiasis and soil-transmitted helminthiasis. Geneva, Switzerland: World Health Organization; 2013.

[27] Cornwell RL, Jones RM. Anthelmintic activity of pyrantel pamoate against *Ancylostoma caninum* in dogs. J Trop Med Hyg 1968;71:165−6.

[28] Desowitz RS, Bell T, Williams J, Cardines R, Tamarua M. Anthelmintic activity of pyrantel pamoate. Am J Trop Med Hyg 1970;19:775−8.

[29] Saif M, Bell WJ, Taha A, Abdel-Meguid M, Abdallah A. Comparison of pyrantel pamoate and bepheniumhydroxynaphthoate in the treatment of *Ancylostoma duodenale* infections. J Egypt Med Assoc 1971;54:791−7.

[30] Villarejos VM, Arguedas-Gamboa JA, Eduarte E, Swartzwelder JC. Experiences with the anthelminthic pyrantel pamoate. Am J Trop Med Hyg 1971;20:842−5.

[31] Bumbalo TS, Fugazzotto DJ, Wyczalek JV. Treatment of enterobiasis with pyrantel-pamoate. Am J Trop Med Hyg 1969;18:50−2.

[32] Seah SKK. Pyrantel pamoate in treatment of helminthiasis in a non-endemic area. Southeast Asian J Trop Med Public Health 1973;4:534−42.

[33] Hsieh H-C, Chen E-R. Treatment of *A. lumbricoides* with small dose of pyrantel pamoate (combantrin). Southeast Asian J Trop Med Public Health 1971;2 362−4.

[34] Cervoni WA, Oliver-González J. Clinical evaluation of pyrantel pamoate in helminthiasis. Am J Trop Med Hyg 1971;20:589−91.

[35] Farahmandian I, Sahba GH, Arfaa F, Jalali H. A comparative evaluation of the therapeutic effect of pyrantel pamoate and bepeniumhydroxynaphthoate on *Ancylostoma duodenale* and other intestinal helminths. J Trop Med Hyg 1972;75:205−7.

[36] Ghadirian E, Sanati A. Preliminary studies on the treatment of hookworm with pyrantel pamoate in Iran. J Trop Med Hyg 1972;75:199−201.

[37] Purnomo, Partono P, Soewarta A. Human intestinal parasites in Karakuak, West Flores, Indonesia and the effect of treatment with mebendazole and pyrantel pamoate. Southeast Asian J Trop Med Public Health 1980;11:324−31.

[38] Imai J, Sakamoto O, Munthe FE, Sinulingga S. Survey for soil-transmitted helminths in Asahan Regency, North Sumatra, Indonesia. Southeast Asian J Trop Med Public Health 1985;16:441−6.

[39] Wang BR, Wang HC, Li LW, Zhang XL, Yue JQ, Wang GX, et al. Comparative efficacy of thienpydin, pyrantel pamoate, mebendazole and albendazole in treating ascariasis and enterobiasis. Chin Med J 1987;100:928−30.

[40] Garcia EG. Treatment of multiple intestinal helminthiasis with oxantel and pyrantel. Drugs 1978;15(Suppl. 1):70−2.

[41] Kale OO. Comparative trial of anthelmintic efficacy of pyrantel pamoate (Combantrin) and thiabendazole (Mintezol). Afr J Med Med Sci 1977;6:89−93.

[42] Janssens PG. Chemotherapy of gastrointestinal nematodiasis in man. In: Vanden Bossche H, Thienpont D, Janssens PG, editors. Chemotherapy of gastrointestinal helminths. Berlin, Heidelberg, Germany: Springer-Verlag; 1985. p. 183−406.

[43] World Health Organization. WHO model list on essential medicines. Geneva, Switzerland: World Health Organization; 2013.

[44] Keiser J, Utzinger J. Efficacy of current drugs against soil-transmitted helminth infections: systematic review and meta-analysis. JAMA 2008;299:1937−48.

[45] Sacko M, De Clercq D, Behnke JM, Gilbert FS, Dorny P, Vercruysse J. Comparison of the efficacy of mebendazole, albendazole and pyrantel in treatment of human hookworm infections in the southern region of Mali, West Africa. Trans R Soc Trop Med Hyg 1999;93:195−203.

[46] Bell WJ, Gould GC. Preliminary report on pyrantel pamoate in the treatment of human hookworm infection. East Afr Med J 1971;48:143−51.

[47] Pandey KN, Sharathchandra SG, Sarin GS, Ajmani NK, Chuttani HK. Pyrantel embonate in treatment of hookworm infestation. Br Med J 1971;4:399−400.

[48] Islam N, Chowdhury NA. Mebendazole and pyrantel pamoate as broad-spectrum anthelmintics. Southeast Asian J Trop Med Public Health 1976;7:81−4.

[49] Farid Z, Bassily S, Miner WF, Hassan A, Laughlin LW. Comparative single/dose treatment of hookworm and roundworm infections with levamisole, pyrantel and bephenium. J Trop Med Hyg 1977;80:107−8.

[50] Griffin L, Okello GB, Pamba HO. Mebendazole: a preliminary study comparing its efficacy against hookworm with pyrantel pamoate (Combantrin) and bephenium hydroxynaphthoate (Alcopar) in patients at Kenyatta National Hospital. East Afr Med J 1982;59:214−19.

[51] Mawdsley JH, Barr RD. Pyrantel pamoate therapy of human hookworm infection in Mauritius. East Afr Med J 1975;52:1−6.

[52] Bell WJ, Nassif S. Field study of pyrantel pamoate in the treatment of mixed roundworm, hookworm and *Trichostrongylus* infections. Am J Trop Med Hyg 1971;20:584−8.

[53] Hsieh H-C, Chen E-R. Treatment of *Ascaris*, hookworm and *Trichuris* in fections with a single dose of pyrantel pamoate (combantrin). Southeast Asian J Trop Med Public Health 1973;4:407−12.

[54] Senewiratne B, Hettiarachchi J, Senewiratne K. A comparative study of the relative efficacy of pyrantel pamoate, bephenium hydroxynaphthoate and tetrachlorethylene in the treatment of *Necator americanus* infection in Ceylon. Ann Trop Med Parasitol 1975;69:233−9.

[55] Choi WY, Lee OR, Lee WK, Kim WK, Chung CS, Ough BO. A clinical trial of oxantel and pyrantel against intestinal nematodes infections. Kisaengchunghak Chapchi 1979;17:60−6.

[56] Botero D, Castaño A. Comparative study of pyrantel pamoate, bephenium hydroxy-naphthoate, and tetrachloroethylene in the treatment of *Necator americanus* infections. Am J Trop Med Hyg 1973;22:45−52.

[57] Kale OO, Bammeke AO, Nwankwo EO. Field trials of pyrantel pamoate (Combantrin) in *Ascaris*, hookworm and *Trichuris* infections. Afr J Med Med Sci 1982;11:23−31.

[58] Kale OO. Controlled comparative study of the efficacy of pyrantel pamoate and a combined regimen of piperazine citrate and bephenium hydroxynaphthoate in the treatment of intestinal nemathelminthiases. Afr J Med Med Sci 1981;10:63−7.

[59] Sinniah B, Sinniah D. The anthelmintic effects of pyrantel pamoate, oxantel-pyrantel pamoate, levamisole and mebendazole in the treatment of intestinal nematodes. Ann Trop Med Parasitol 1981;75:315−21.

[60] Sinniah B, Sinniah D, Dissanaike AS. Single dose treatment of intestinal nematodes with oxantel-pyrantel pamoate plus mebendazole. Ann Trop Med Parasitol 1980;74:619−23.

[61] World Health Organisation. Controlling disease due to soil-transmitted helminths. Geneva, Switzerland: World Health Organization; 2003.

[62] Hong S-T, Chai J-Y, Choi M-H, Huh S, Rim HJ, Lee SH. A successful experience of soil-transmitted helminth control in the Republic of Korea. Korean J Parasitol 2006;44:177−85.

[63] Keiser J, Utzinger J. The drugs we have and the drugs we need against major hel-minth infections. Adv Parasitol 2010;73:197−230.

[64] Olliaro P, Seiler J, Kuesel A, Horton J, Clark JN, Don R, et al. Potential drug devel-opment candidates for human soil-transmitted helminthiases. PLoS Negl Trop Dis 2011;5:e1138.

[65] Smith G. A mathematical model for the evolution of anthelmintic resistance in a direct life cycle nematode parasite. Int J Parasitol 1990;20:913−21.

[66] Barnes EH, Dobson RJ, Barger IA. Worm control and anthelmintic resistance: adventures with a model. Parasitol Today 1995;11:56−63.

[67] Leathwick DM. Modelling the benefits of releasing a new class of anthelmintic in combination. Vet Parasitol 2012;186:93−100.

[68] Bartram DJ, Leathwick DM, Taylor MA, Geurden T, Maeder SJ. The role of com-bination anthelmintic formulations in the sustainable control of sheep nematodes. Vet Parasitol 2012;186:151−8.

[69] Leathwick DM, Waghorn TS, Miller CM, Candy PM, Oliver AM. Managing anthelmintic resistance-use of a combination anthelmintic and leaving some lambs untreated to slow the development of resistance to ivermectin. Vet Parasitol 2012;187:285−94.

[70] Knopp SR, Kotze AC, McCarthy JS, Coleman GT. High-level pyrantel resistance in the hookworm *Ancylostoma caninum*. Vet Parasitol 2007;143:299−304.

[71] Roepstorff A, Bjørn H, Nansen P. Resistance of *Oesphagostomum* spp. in pigs to pyrantel citrate. Vet Parasitol 1987;24:229−39.

[72] Coles GC, Brown SN, Trembath CM. Pyrantel-resistant large strongyles in racehorses. Vet Record 1999;145:408.

[73] Kaplan RM, Klei TR, Lyons ET, Lester G, Courtney CH, French DD, et al. Anthelmintic resistant cyathostomes on horse farms. J Am Vet Med Assoc 2004;225:903—10.

[74] Meier A, Hertzberg H. Equine strongyles II. Occurrence of anthelmintic resistance in Switzerland. Schweizer Archiv fur Tierhelk 2005;148:389—96.

[75] Reynoldson J, Behnke J, Pallant L, MacnishM, Gilbert F, Giles S, et al. Failure of pyrantel in treatment of human hookworm infections (Ancylostoma duodenale) in the Kimberley region of North West Australia. Acta Tropica 1997;68:301—12.

[76] Albonico M, Bickle Q, Ramsan M, Montresor A, Savioli L, Taylor M. Efficacy of mebendazole and levamisole alone or in combination against intestinal nematode infections after repeated targeted mebendazole treatment in Zanzibar. Bull World Health Organ 2003;81:343—52.

[77] Beach MJ, Streit TG, Addiss DG, Prospere R, Roberts JM, Lammie PJ. Assessment of combined ivermectin and albendazole for treatment of intestinal helminth and Wuchereria bancrofti infections in Haitian school children. Am J Trop Med Hyg 1999;60:479—86.

[78] Ismail MM, Jayakody RL. Efficacy of albendazole and its combinations with iver-mectin or diethylcarbamazine (DEC) in the treatment of Trichuris trichiura infections in Sri Lanka. Ann Trop Med Parasitol 1999;93:501—4.

[79] Belizario VY, Amarillo ME, de Leon WU, de los Reyes AE, Bugayong MG, Macatangay BJ. A comparison of the efficacy of single doses of albendazole, iver-mectin, and diethylcarbamazine alone or in combinations against Ascaris and Trichuris spp. Bull World Health Organ 2003;81:35—42.

[80] Ndyomugyenyi R, Kabatereine N, Olsen A, Magnussen P. Efficacy of ivermectin and albendazole alone and in combination for treatment of soil-transmitted hel-minths in pregnancy and adverse events: a randomized open label controlled inter-vention trial in Masindi district, western Uganda. Am J Trop Med Hyg 2008;79:856—63.

[81] Knopp S, Mohammed KA, Speich B, Hattendorf J, Khamis IS, Khamis AN, et al. Albendazole and mebendazole administered alone or in combination with ivermec-tin against Trichuris trichiura: a randomized controlled trial. Clin Infect Dis 2010;51:1420—8.

[82] Speich B, Ali SM, Ame SM, Alles R, Huwyler J, Albonico M, et al. Efficacy and safety of albendazole plus ivermectin, albendazole plus mebendazole, albendazole plus oxantel, pamoate, and mebendazole alone against Trichuris trichiura and concom-itant soil-transmitted helminth infections: a four-arm, randomised controlled trial. Lancet Infect Dis 2015;15:277—84.

[83] Speich B, Ame SM, Ali SM, Alles R, Hattendorf J, Utzinger J, et al. Efficacy and safety of nitazoxanide, albendazole, and nitazoxanide-albendazole against Trichuris tri-chiura infection: a randomized controlled trial. PLoS Negl Trop Dis 2012;6:e1685.

[84] Speich B, Ame SM, Ali SM, Alles R, Huwyler J, Hattendorf J, et al. Oxantel pamoate-albendazole for Trichuris trichiura infection. N Engl J Med 2014;370:610—20.

CHAPTER 6

Potential Applications of Tetrahydropyrimidines to Address Unmet Needs

A.A. Marchiondo[1,2]

[1]Adobe Veterinary Parasitology Consulting LLC, Santa Fe, NM, United States
[2]Retired, Zoetis, Kalamazoo, MI, United States

6.1 EXPANDED LABEL CLAIMS IN EQUINE COMBINATIONS—TAPEWORM ACTIVITY

Once a new anthelmintic class or compound has been discovered in the animal health industry, extensive in vitro and in vivo studies are conducted to determine the full spectrum of anthelmintic activity. The positive and negative results of these dose determination studies serve to identify those animal species and markets, for example, companion animal, cattle, etc., for which the compound will be formulated and developed for commercialization. All potential anthelmintic activities against numerous parasite species within hosts may be explored during the product development process. However, not all anthelmintic activities are pursued as specific label claims for product registration against a particular stage or species of parasite. A case in point is the activity of pyrantel pamoate against *Anoplocephala perfoliata* at the dosage of 13.2 mg/kg body weight (b.w.).

Pyrantel pamoate administered at the recommended nematocidal dose of 6.6 mg pyrantel base/kg b.w. has shown partial cestocidal activity of 0–100%, with average efficacies of 70–87% against *A. perfoliata* [1–4]. At the elevated (2X) dose of 13.2 mg pyrantel base/kg b.w., pyrantel pamoate has exhibited 93–97.8% efficacy against *A. perfoliata* [4–7]. Thus, the dose of 13.2 mg pyrantel base/kg b.w. (ie, doubling the nematocidal single dose) has become a widely accepted target dose for treating *A. perfoliata* infections in horses.

Although the labels of some European paste formulations of pyrantel embonate listed *A. perfoliata*, the tapeworm dosage was never an approved dose level by the regulatory authorities in the United States, as the necessary studies for label claim approval were never conducted. It was not until April 18, 2005 that Supplemental NADA 200-342 was approved by the FDA/CVM for administration as a single oral dose of 6 mg pyrantel base per pound of body weight (13.2 mg/kg b.w.) for treatment of tapeworms (*A. perfoliata*). This regulatory approval came only after the completion of dose confirmation studies (efficacies of 95.5−98.4% [8]), field studies (efficacies of 92−98%, overall 95% [9]), and target animal safety studies to verify the efficacy and safety of pyrantel pamoate at 13.2 mg/kg b.w. [10]. At the present time, pyrantel pamoate at 13.2 mg/kg b.w. offers an alternative to praziquantel [11] as an efficacious and safe treatment of *A. perfoliata* in horses. While there are equine combination products that include praziquantel to treat tapeworms in horses, no equine combination has been developed and approved with pyrantel pamoate to treat *A. perfoliata*.

6.2 COMBINATION APPLICATIONS AGAINST RESISTANT PARASITES—EQUINE

Anthelmintic resistance is becoming increasingly prevalent among equine nematode parasites [12]. Emerging macrocyclic lactone (ML) resistance to ivermectin or moxidectin in certain isolates of *Parascaris equorum* was first reported from the Netherlands [13] and Canada [14] after treatment at the recommended dosages failed to reduce ascarid egg counts. Subsequently, isolated populations of *P. equorum* resistant to MLs have been reported from the United States [15,16], Denmark [17], Germany [18], the Netherlands [19], Brazil [20], Sweden [21], and Italy [22]. While initial reports were based on the failure of ML treatment to reduce fecal egg counts, an efficacy study with artificially infected foals unequivocally confirmed resistance when ivermectin treatment (200 µg/kg b.w.) reduced adult ascarid numbers by only 22% [23]. Resistance to MLs clearly involves both ivermectin and moxidectin because sequential dosing of individual foals with ivermectin and moxidectin failed to reduce egg counts after either treatment [24].

Pyrantel pamoate, fenbendazole, and oxibendazole have been used successfully in the field to treat ML-resistant populations of ascarids [14−17, 25], but those reports were based on fecal egg count reduction testing. Accordingly, a definitive efficacy evaluation with a paste formulation of pyrantel pamoate (13.2 mg/kg b.w.) using foals that had been artificially infected with a known ML-resistant isolate of *P. equorum* demonstrated 97.3% efficacy [26].

Along with the ML-resistance reports emerging against the equine asca- rid, putative failures after anthelmintic treatment to remove adult pinworm (*Oxyuris equi*) infections have been reported by numerous practitioners. Although some perceived failures were based on persistent anal pruritus after anthelmintic treatment, a portion of these reports included unequivocal evi- dence of pinworm survival, such as passage of adult worms in feces several weeks after treatment, or appearance of typical egg masses in the perianal region. Most anecdotal reports of treatment failure have involved the repeated use of ivermectin in mature horses. ML resistance in adult pin- worms *O. equi* in the United States has been reported with pinworm infec- tions surviving ivermectin treatment at the label dosage of 200 µg/kg b.w. [27]. Pinworms surviving ivermectin treatment were subsequently removed by pyrantel pamoate paste (6.6 mg/kg b.w.), suggesting that some individual nematodes within the population were not uniformly susceptible to ML anthelmintics. Other researchers in the United States have reported the sur- vival of ivermectin treatment by adult and larval pinworms [28], but some putative ML-resistant pinworm populations have been shown to be fully sus- ceptible to ivermectin [29]. The possible development of resistance to MLs in equine oxyurosis has been reported in two cases in Germany with anthel- mintic failure of moxidectin and ivermectin resulting in persistent *O. equi* infections with continuous egg shedding [30].

The efficacies of pyrantel pamoate against ML-resistant *P. equorum* and *O. equi* are further examples of anthelmintic activities that might be exploited in an ML + pyrantel pamoate combination formulation. This strategy confers advantages [31,32] that include, but are not limited, to (1) controlling ML-resistant nematodes, and (2) limiting/preventing the selection pressure of ML- and pyrantel-resistance, thus preserving the use- fulness of both anthelmintics. The granting of regulatory label claims against resistant isolates of nematodes in companion animals and food- producing animals has not occurred in the United States, unlike Australia. From a marketing standpoint, a label claim for a product against a nema- tode isolate resistant to a competitor molecule would be considered highly valuable in the market place.

REFERENCES

[1] Lyons ET, Drudge JH, Tolliver SC. Critical tests of three salts of pyrantel against internal parasites of the horse. Am J Vet Res 1974;35:1515−22.
[2] Slocombe JOD. Prevalence and treatment of tapeworms in horses. Can Vet J 1979;20:136−40.

[3] Lyons ET, Drudge JH, Tolliver SC, Swerczek TW, Collins SS. Determination of the efficacy of pyrantel pamoate at the therapeutic dose rate against the tapeworm *Anoplocephala perfoliata* in equids using a modification of the critical test method. Vet Parasitol 1989;31(1):13–18.

[4] Lyons ET, Tolliver SC, Drudge JH. Further evaluation of pyrantel pamoate at the therapeutic dose rate (6.6 mg base/kg) against *Anoplocephala perfoliata* in horses. J Helminthol Soc Wash 1997;64:285–7.

[5] Lyons ET, Drudge JH, Tolliver SC. Pyrantel pamoate: evaluating its activity against equine tapeworms. Vet Med 1986;81:280–5.

[6] Slocombe JOD, De Gannes R, Lake M. Effectiveness of pyrantel pamoate for *Parascaris* resistant to macrocyclic lactones [abstract]. Proc 49th AAVP/79th ASP 2004;49:46 2004.

[7] Höglund J, Nilsson O, Ljunström BL, Hellander J, Lind EO, Uggla A. Epidemiology of *Anoplocephala perfoliata* infection in foals on a stud farm in southwestern Sweden. Vet Parasitol 1989;75(1):71–9.

[8] Reinemeyer CR, Hutchens DE, Eckblad WP, Marchiondo AA, Shugart JI. Dose-confirmation studies of the cestocidal activity of pyrantel pamoate paste in horses. Vet Parasitol 2006;138:234–9.

[9] Marchiondo AA, White GW, Smith LL, Reinemeyer CR, Dascanio JJ, Johnson EG, et al. Clinical field efficacy and safety of pyrantel pamoate paste (19.13% w/w pyrantel base) against *Anoplocephala* spp. in naturally infected horses. Vet. Parasitol. 2006;137:94–102.

[10] Marchiondo AA, TerHune TN, Herrick RL. Target animal safety and tolerance study of pyrantel pamoate paste (19.13% w/w pyrantel base) orally administered to horses. Vet. Ther 2005;6(4):301–14.

[11] Coles GC, Hillyer MH, Taylor FG, Villard I. Efficacy of an ivermectin-praziquantel combination in equids against bots and tapeworms. Vet Rec 2003;152(6):178–9.

[12] Nielsen MK, Reinemeyer CR, Donecker JM, Leathwick DM, Marchiondo AA, Kaplan RM. Anthelmintic resistance in equine parasites-current evidence and knowledge gaps. Vet Parasitol 2014;204(1-2):55–63.

[13] Boersema JH, Eysker M, Nas JW. Apparent resistance of *Parascaris* equorum to macrocyclic lactones. Vet Rec 2002;150:279–81.

[14] Hearn FP, Peregrine AS. Identification of foals infected with *Parascaris equorum* apparently resistant to ivermectin. J Am Vet Med Assoc 2003;223:482–5.

[15] Craig TM, Diamond PL, Ferwerda NS, Thompson. Evidence of ivermectin resistance by *Parascaris equorum* on a Texas horse farm. J Equine Vet Sci 2007;27:67–71.

[16] Lyons ET, Tolliver SC, Ionita M, Collins SS. Evaluation of parasiticidal activity of fenbendazole, ivermectin, oxibendazole, and pyrantel pamoate in horse foals with emphasis on ascarids (*Parascaris equorum*) in field studies on five farms in Central Kentucky in 2007. Parasitol Res 2008;103:287–91.

[17] Schougaard H, Nielsen MK. Apparent ivermectin resistance of *Parascaris equorum* in foals in Denmark. Vet Rec 2007;160:439–40.

[18] von Samson-Himmelstjerna G, Fritzen B, Demeler J, Schurmann S, Rohn K, Schnieder T, et al. Cases of reduced cyathostomin egg-reappearance period and failure of *Parascaris equorum* egg count reduction following ivermectin treatment as well as survey on pyrantel efficacy on German horse farms. Vet Parasitol 2007;144:74–80.

[19] van Doorn D.C.K., Lems S., Weteling A., Ploeger H.W., Eysker M. Resistance of *Parascaris equorum* against ivermectin due to frequent anthelmintic treatment of foals in the Netherlands. In: Proc World Assoc Adv Vet Parasitol 21st international conference; 19–23 August, 2007. p. 133.

[20] Molento M, Antunes J, Bentes RN. Anthelmintic resistance in Brazilian horses. Vet Rec 2008;162:384—5.
[21] Lindgren K, Ljungvall Ö, Nilsson O, Ljungström BL, Lindahl C, Höglund J. *Parascaris equorum* in foals and in their environment on a Swedish stud farm, with notes on treatment failure of ivermectin. Vet Parasitol 2008;151:337—43.
[22] Veronesi F, Moretta I, Moretti A, Fioretti DP, Genchi C. Field effectiveness of pyrantel and failure of *Parascaris equorum* egg count reduction following ivermectin treatment in Italian horse farms. Vet Parasitol 2009;161:138—41.
[23] Kaplan R.M., Reinemeyer C.R., Slocombe J.O., Murray M.J. Confirmation of ivermectin resistance in a purportedly resistant Canadian isolate of *Parascaris equorum* in foals. In: Proc Am Assoc Vet Parasitol 2006 51st annual meeting; 15—18 July 2006. pp. 69—70.
[24] Reinemeyer C.R., Marchiondo A.A. Efficacy of pyrantel pamoate in horses against a macrocyclic lactone-resistant isolate of *Parascaris equorum*. In: Proc Am Assoc Vet Parasitol 52nd annual meeting; 14—17 July, 2007. p. 78.
[25] Slocombe JOD, de Gannes RV, Lake MC. Macrocyclic lactone-resistant *Parascaris equorum* on stud farms in Canada and effectiveness of fenbendazole and pyrantel pamoate. Vet Parasitol 2007;145:371—6.
[26] Reinemeyer CR, Prado JC, Nichols EC, Marchiondo AA. Efficacy of pyrantel pamoate against a macrocyclic lactone-resistant isolate of *Parasacris equorum* in horses. Vet Parasitol 2010;171:111—15.
[27] Reinemeyer C.R., Marchiondo A.A., Shugart J.I. Macrocyclic lactone-resistant *Oxyuris equi*: anecdote or emerging problem? In: Proc Am Assoc Vet Parasitol 51st annual meeting; 15—19, July 2006b. p. 67.
[28] Lyons E, Tolliver S, Collins S. Probable reason why small strongyle EPG counts are returning "early" after ivermectin treatment of horses on a farm in Central Kentucky. Parasitol Res 2009;104:569—74.
[29] Reinemeyer CR, Prado JC, Nichols EC, Marchiondo AA. Efficacy of pyrantel pamoate and ivermectin paste formulations against naturally acquired *Oxyuris equi* in horses. Vet Parasitol 2010;171:106—10.
[30] Wolf DC, Hermosilla C, Taubert A. *Oxyuris equi*: lack of efficacy in treatment with macrocyclic lactones. Vet Parasitol 2014;201(1-2):163—8.
[31] Leathwick DM, Hosking BC. Managing anthelmintic resistance: modeling strategic use of a new anthelmintic class to slow the development of resistance to existing classes. N Z Vet J 2009;57(4):203—7.
[32] Leathwick DM, Besier RB. The management of anthelmintic resistance in grazing ruminants in Australasia—strategies and experiences. Vet Parasitol 2014;204:44—54.

INDEX

Note: Page numbers followed by "*f*" and "*t*" refer to figures and tables, respectively.

Printed in the United States
By Bookmasters